Caring for People in Pain

This book is about good practice in the care of people in pain. Drugs, physical and psycho-social interventions all have their part to play in helping the person in pain, but the way in which care is delivered is equally important.

Caring for People in Pain is divided into four parts. The first sets the scene and demonstrates the different kinds of pain with which the practitioner may be faced. The second looks in detail at the factors involved in the experience of pain, and clearly explains the function of neuro-physiological mechanisms and the importance of Gate Control Theory. The author then goes on to look at the role of emotion and cognition in creating meaning and defining the experience of pain. The final section of the second part looks at the social and cultural factors which lead to different ways of coping with pain and which influence the response to various interventions. The third part considers the different types of intervention available to the practitioner, both physical and psychological, and in the fourth and final part the role of the nurse is shown to be crucial in managing the patient's experience of pain.

This evidence-based guide to good practice in pain management provides a comprehensive and accessible text for students on all entry-level and many post-registration nursing courses.

Bryn D. Davis is Head of Department of Nursing Studies and Dean of School of Nursing, University of Wales College of Medicine, Cardiff.

Routledge Essentials for Nurses cover four key areas of nursing:

- core theoretical studies
- psychological and physical care
- nurse education
- new directions in nursing and health care

Written by experienced practitioners and teachers, books in this series encourage a critical approach to nursing concepts and show how research findings are relevant to nursing practice.

The series editors are **Robert Newell**, University of Leeds and **David Thompson**, University of York and Nursing Advisor at the Department of Health.

Also in this series:

Nursing Theories and Models   Hugh McKenna
Nursing Perspectives on Quality of Life   Peter Draper
Education for Patients and Clients   Vivien Coates

Caring for People
in Pain

Bryn D. Davis

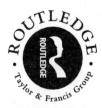

London and New York

First published 2000
by Routledge
11 New Fetter Lane, London EC4P 4EE

Simultaneously published in the USA and Canada
by Routledge
29 West 35th Street, New York, NY 10001

Routledge is an imprint of the Taylor & Francis Group

© 2000 Bryn D. Davis

Typeset in Times by Taylor & Francis Books Ltd
Printed and bound in Great Britain by MPG Books Ltd, Bodmin

British Library Cataloguing in Publication Data
A catalogue record for this book is available from the British
Library

Library of Congress Cataloging in Publication Data
Davis, Bryn D.
   Caring for People in Pain / Bryn D. Davis
   Includes bibliographical references and index.
   1. Pain – Nursing. 2. Pain – Treatment. I. Title.
   RT87.P35.D38   2000   99–36130
   616'.0472–dc21   CIP

ISBN 0–415–18890–3 (hbk)
ISBN 0–415–18891–1 (pbk)

Contents

Illustrations

Figures

Boxes

Acknowledgements

I should like to acknowledge the help I continue to receive from my colleagues in the nursing world of pain: from my research students, Pat Schofield, Jane Latham, Trudy Towell, Angeliki Dreliozi, and Clare Herbert; and from Meg Gorman, Liz Morgan and colleagues in the TDS branch of the University of Wales College of Medicine Library.

My wife Catherine, and children Sarah and Robert have been most patient and supportive during the many months of preparation of this volume; to them it is dedicated.

Part 1

Introduction

What is pain?

Chapter 1

Introduction

The 'inside story'

There has been a great deal of development in the understanding of the pain experience over the last forty years or so and particularly over the last ten to fifteen. The pace of research and development seems even to be increasing. The kind of picture that we now have of the kinds of experiences people have when they are in pain, and the mechanisms that help to bring those experiences about, is very complex. It involves all aspects of our nature from our physiology and biochemistry to our emotional and motivational make up, to our psychological processes and being, to our social relationships and to our sense of spiritual awareness.

In attempting to help people in pain it is most important that we understand that complexity and that, in our assessments of need, and planning of care, we incorporate that range of knowledge and insight. Each of the facets mentioned above does not act in isolation, but as part of an interacting dynamic whole. When someone experiences pain, their whole being can be involved, and we can use aspects of that whole being to help them, and to help them to help themselves.

The experience of pain is essentially an individual, internal experience, known only to the person with the pain. We who try to help them come to it very much from the outside. What we know of it is what we can learn from that person. This knowledge can, of course, add up to a lot of general insights into pain, but each person's experience is different, and personal. The purpose of this book then is to try to demonstrate that 'inside story' of pain. The mechanisms and processes, at physiological/biochemical, emotional/motivational, cognitive/evaluative and social/cultural levels will be considered to present a holistic view. It is hoped that those caring for people in pain will be able to gain insight into the individual's own experience and to develop a plan of care that meets those individual needs.

Who is this book for?

This book is aimed at those practitioners who are involved in caring for people in pain. Primarily this means nurses. However, there are other health-care professionals involved in this area, and it is hoped that they might also find the volume useful.

The main focus of the book is on the needs of the undergraduate pre-registration student. However, there are many registered nurses who are involved in the management of pain who wish to update their knowledge. They might be undertaking a post-registration degree or even a master's level study of pain. It is hoped that the level of the book will meet the needs of these different groups. Even if not undertaking a formal course it is hoped that the practising nurse will be able to access the information here in order to enhance her or his practice.

Why do we need this book?

One of the main reasons for this book is the continuing evidence for poor pain management. This is associated with the continuing existence of many myths and misconceptions about the pain experience and its care (e.g. IASP 1992; McCaffrey et al. 1994). There is evidence for poor pain assessment (Seers 1987; Paice et al. 1991), the under or over assessment of pain by staff (Carr 1990; Zalon 1993) and failure to prescribe or administer enough analgesics (Bonica 1980; Donovan et al. 1987; Closs 1990; Paice et al. 1991). This applies also and particularly to children and infants (Mather and Mackie 1983; Beyer and Byers 1985; Carr 1990; Gonzalez et al. 1993; Carter 1994).

Poor levels of knowledge have been identified as an important aspect (Sofaer 1984; Watt-Watson 1987; Fothergill-Bourbonnais and Wilson-Barnett 1992; McCaffrey et al. 1994). This applies to nurses in a variety of settings. These results also demonstrate a failure to improve the situation over a long period.

The knowledgeable carer

In order to address this latter factor of poor knowledge and to facilitate educational developments for nurses and other health-care professionals, this volume has been written with a particular approach which it is felt has not been offered before. The emphasis is more on the experience of being in pain and how this should influence the care given to those in pain. Thus from an exploration of the factors influencing the experience of pain, and the way that the experience of pain can vary from individual to individual, an approach to care will be advocated that should lead to more effective management of pain. In this way the practitioner should therefore be able to claim to be offering a more caring role to those in pain.

By caring is meant a more considerate role; an approach that is much more concerned with the needs of the individual, but one that shows a much more understanding, empathetic relationship with the sufferer. It also benefits from insights gained from an understanding of the factors and mechanisms that can operate on and within individuals. These include the physical, emotional, cognitive, social and cultural factors (Leininger 1991; Morse 1995, cited in McKenna 1997). It includes the desire to work *with* the individual in pain, rather than a desire to do things *to* or *for* him or her (Gazda *et al.* 1987). This will then lead to the development of a very individualised plan which when implemented will show care.

In many ways then this book is not so much about nociception, that is, the transmission of noxious stimuli from the periphery to the central nervous system. It is more about what factors or processes lead to a particular experience, by an individual, that leads to the claim that he or she is in pain. From an understanding of these, and the development of skills in assessing these individual processes and factors, the nurse or other health-care professional will be in a position to help in the management of that pain.

Diamond and Coniam (1991) argue that the pain experience arises from the functioning of both the body and the mind. This insight reflects a long history in attempts to understand it (see Merskey 1980). Others, for example Cassel (1991), have argued that we should incorporate the concept of suffering as well because in some pain experiences it is difficult to specify a particular pain as the experience is more holistic and thus justifies the term suffering rather than pain.

As a student the reader is expected to incorporate the information in this book into their developing practice. It should be read in conjunction with other reference texts, such as those in psychology and sociology, as well as pharmacology, anatomy, physiology and biochemistry. As a staff nurse or other practitioner, the reader is expected to draw on his or her experience and previous reading to place this volume in context.

The structure of the book

The book is organised into parts. The first part sets the scene, and describes the different kinds of pain with which the practitioner might be faced. This is particularly aimed at the relative newcomer so that lack of experience should not prevent a proper understanding of the information in the book. However, it is hoped that the more experienced practitioner may come across some different aspects of pain from those with which they are familiar or at least be able to confirm their experience, in the examples given.

The second part is perhaps the main part. In these four chapters the nature of the pain experience and in particular the 'inside story' is explored. By this is meant the range of factors, including peripheral nociception, but certainly not exclusively, that lead to a painful experience. Certainly the neuro-physiological mechanisms will be considered and of course the importance of the Gate Control Theory offered by Melzack and Wall (1965) in explaining the processes that seem to produce that painful feeling. It is from this theory that the particular approach taken in this volume is taken.

However, a more substantial part of this second part will cover the emotional, motivational, and cognitive-evaluative aspects of the pain experience. As well as receiving information coming in from the periphery, the central nervous system and its cognitive, emotional, experiencing functions are creating meanings and defining experiences. These are related to any incoming information but not necessarily directly and sometimes without any apparent relationship.

As well as these emotional, motivational and cognitive-evaluative factors and processes, social and cultural factors will be explored. Through these the individual learns patterns of behaviour or of thought and feeling that influence the kind of meaning and definition that he or she will put on any experience. These will in their turn lead to forms of expression of the experience that will vary from individual to individual or from time to time in the same individual. These forms of expression will also include ways of coping (or not coping) with the pain. They will also influence the reaction or response to various interventions that may be offered or applied to prevent or treat the pain.

In Part III these various interventions will be considered. It is from a study of the factors and processes involved in the pain experience of any individual that we can gain a proper understanding of how interventions might work or how they might best be used. They will include the traditional pharmacological preparations that have been and continue to be developed and refined to help people cope with pain. These are of course an important aspect of the management of pain. However, in many instances they are not as successful as might be wished, or they lose their efficacy over time.

This then leads to the study of other complementary or alternative approaches which can involve both physical and psycho-social measures. There are a variety of physical interventions, including electrical, heat and cold, massage and aromatics, and counter-irritation. However, there are also many interventions based on psychology that can help to prevent pain or to enable the sufferer to develop meanings for the pain that give him or her a greater sense of control over the situation. Other psychologically based approaches include relaxation and distraction.

Also included in this important part are other approaches derived from other models of health and illness, perhaps from different cultures. They include acupuncture and herbal medicine. With many of these interventions there is a great opportunity for nurses and other health-care professionals to develop their relationship with the patient. In this way they can become more of a partner with him or her, allowing the sufferer a much more important, perhaps leading, role in the management of their pain.

In the final part the role of the nurse in particular is considered. The nurse of course is a member of a multi-professional team and as such must be aware of the various parts that can be played by each of the professions involved. A particular aspect of the management of the patient's experience of pain is that of the assessment of that experience. The patient is the only person who can do this and the role of the nurse or other professional is to help the sufferer express adequately the nature and intensity of the pain so that suitable and adequate interventions may be proposed and implemented. As well as assessing the pain there is an important role in the regular monitoring of the effectiveness or otherwise of any interventions that might be implemented. In this way modifications to the interventions or alternatives may be introduced.

Nurses have a very important role in the administration of many of the interventions, and particularly in information giving and education. Other health-care professionals may also be involved here and it is important that the team agree as to who is to be responsible for what activity so that there is no unnecessary repetition and there are no gaps. Many nurses have developed specialist roles regarding the management of pain and there are now many pain clinics where specialist teams are employed. Some of these deal only with certain kinds of pain or with special client groups, in the hospital setting or in the patient's own home or in hospices, as part of palliative care.

In the final chapter there will be a summary of what has gone before, and a discussion as to where the care of people in pain should be going in the future. It is important that education, at both pre- and post-registration levels, is developed, and that nurses, and other professionals, recognise the need for regular updating, of knowledge, attitudes and skills. The utilisation of research in practice, so that more clinically effective care is available to people in pain, is a professional responsibility. Also, there is still much more research needed, not only into various mechanisms of the pain experience but also into interventions or even the management and administration of the interventions that we have. It is in this way through research and development that a more personalised, caring and effective approach to helping the sufferer may be achieved.

The evaluation of current and new methods of helping people in pain is all part of the ongoing management of care and of the accountability of the professional. The purpose of this book is to help the professional to be aware of the processes and factors involved, of the research that gives us this information and the practices that are based on this research. With all the information available today there is little need for any person to be in unmanaged pain. Yet there is recent evidence that this does still occur, in the acute and the chronic situation, with the very young and with the elderly. This evidence will be considered in more detail in a later chapter dealing with pain management. It is mentioned here to remind the reader of the importance of the study of ways of caring for people in pain.

Chapter 2

Some experiences of pain

> The least pain in our little finger gives us more concern and uneasiness than the destruction of millions of our fellow-beings.
>
> William Hazlitt

Introduction

The main focus of this volume is the experience of people in pain. It is an attempt to explore the kinds of experiences that sufferers have, and the factors and processes that create the experience that sufferers call pain.

For professionals there is a tendency to see or approach pain from the outside of the sufferer, in terms of tissue damage, and neuro-physiological processes. Indeed many professionals seem to have their own views as to what is allowed to be called pain, and when any intervention might be necessary (McCaffrey *et al.* 1994).

Yet pain can be seen as being essentially 'all in the mind', being the interpretation by the sufferer of information coming from the peripheral nervous system (which may also include internal parts, such as the abdomen, thorax, cranium and the spine), into the cortex and related emotional centres. The interpretation is influenced by physical, psychological and socio-cultural factors and processes. As some definitions have it, it is what the patient says it is and occurs when the patient says it does (e.g. McCaffrey 1968). Other definitions try to incorporate some indication of the link with tissue damage (e.g. Sternbach 1968; Mountcastle 1980; Merskey 1986). This latter is one that is frequently referenced in other texts. However, Melzack and Wall (1996) discuss this question of definitions and find it difficult to accept in its entirety any of these. They argue that pain research has not yet developed to a level at which it is possible to give a definition from which practice, education and research can develop. Pain can mean so many things to so many different people that we must be careful in tying ourselves down to a particular definition yet.

There is, of course, often tissue damage present in some obvious form to 'explain' or justify the claim of being in pain by the sufferer. Nevertheless the pain sometimes is reported when the tissue damage seems to have been repaired, or to be out of proportion to the apparent damage. There are instances of what is called 'central pain' whereby there is no apparent peripheral source of the pain, or of pain being reported in relation to non-existent parts of the body, such as an amputated limb. There are also some relatively rare examples of no pain being reported when there is apparent tissue damage (Melzack and Wall 1996).

In this chapter we shall present and discuss some of these different types of pain experience in an attempt to get 'inside' the patient/sufferer's experience. There have been several attempts to classify types of pain, based on a variety of sources of information, for example that of P. A. McGrath (1990) in which pain is classified into acute, chronic, recurrent and cancer. With a cluster analysis of patients' scores on SCR-90R scales, Williams *et al.* (1995) found three groups involving both men and women. Sub-group one had much psychological distress, and also the highest levels of pain and depression. Sub-group two had lower levels of psychological distress and pain, and high levels of depression and somatisation. Sub-group three had least pain and least depression. In another cluster analysis, Tait and Chibnall (1998) studied attitudes to pain of patients. They identified two main groups: one displayed self-reliant attitude sets; the other demonstrated medically orientated attitudes. Both main groups had sub-groups, one of which demonstrated little emotionality associated with the pain and the other high levels of emotionality.

Turk and Melzack (1992) have discussed extensively the question of the classification of pain and find many different ways of achieving this. They have explored behavioural, cognitive-psychological, empirical, multi-dimensional and clustering methods. They come to the conclusion that different types of classification systems should be used in the clinical setting so that communication and understanding can be evaluated. This might then enable us to deal on a more individual basis with our patients and clients (Turk and Rudy 1990). For the purposes of this volume however a simple system of classification has been developed to facilitate the discussion of the different aspects of the pain experience. This is: pain on injury (including surgery); pain from disease (acute); pain from disease (chronic); and unusual pain situations (see Box 2.1).

Box 2.1   Types of pain

Pain on injury (including surgery)	bruising; sprain; broken bone; surgical pain
Pain from disease (acute)	MI; cholecystitis; toothache; migraine (headache); appendicitis
Pain from disease (chronic)	cancer pain; arthritis; low back pain
Unusual pain situations	inability to communicate; phantom limb pain; inability to feel pain

---

Pain on injury (including surgery)

Most people experience some form of injury during their lives. Even, and perhaps in particular, in childhood we are subject to bumps and bruises, cuts and sprains as a result of exploring our world and in taking part in sport or other physical activities. More rarely one may experience a broken bone or more serious laceration of tissue in a major accident. Cycle and road accidents are frequent occasions for experiencing pain.

In these situations the pain is usually very intense, localised to the site of the injury, and leads to identification of the cause and the search for treatment. We tend not to want to use or move the part, as in the case of a bad bruise or sprain. The sharp, intense feeling of pain may be mixed up with aches and feelings of soreness around the site of intensity. Alternatively the pain may feel 'deep' or be described by the sufferer as 'shooting' or 'stabbing'. There may be feelings of tissues being stretched or bursting or burning. There may be a sense of pressure, pressing inwards or outwards. This is usually associated with the inflammatory response to the injury (Rang and Bevan 1994).

In many ways the pain associated with injury can be explained or understood as a result of the damage caused. Occasionally there is pain from an injury that is not visible which may be difficult to understand. There is always an emotional reaction to pain, even when obvious and understandable, but the fear and uncertainty of invisible injury may make the experience even more traumatic (Johnston 1980; Seers 1987; Poole 1998). Some people can respond in a very extreme way and feel that the end of the world has come, that nothing worse can ever happen to them ('catastrophisers', Skevington 1995; Melzack and Wall 1996).

Shock is often a psycho-physiological response to injury and severe pain (Boore *et al.* 1987). Here the mind and body seem to suffer a generalised reaction, which involves reduced blood pressure, dizziness, fainting or even unconsciousness. As well as being a response to the amount of tissue damage, the loss of blood or other body fluids, shock can also be a reaction to the intensity of the pain itself. The patient feels weak, dizzy, there may be nausea and vomiting. There is difficulty in concentrating, in thinking, so that the victim is relatively unable to help themselves or to give a clear picture as to what has happened or what they are experiencing. There may be loss of memory of the event itself although this is usually short term. To a certain extent this period in shock will tend to cloud the experience of pain, and little or none may be reported.

The situation in accident and emergency departments can provide many examples of this as can the immediate post-operative experience (Carr and Thomas 1997; Herbert 1998). As the patient recovers from the shock (often with the help of IV fluids, rest and warmth as well as psychological reassurance and explanation) then the experience of pain will become more real, and more clearly experienced and expressed.

Pain from surgery

Surgery can be seen as an intentional injury, whereby particular tissues and organs of the body are cut or reshaped or removed in order to overcome disease or to help the body to recover from some accidental injury. Some surgical interventions are for psychological or cosmetic purposes, or to straighten or repair deformed parts.

The pain involved can to a large extent be anticipated and planned for. In most cases there should be little or no pain experienced. Modern techniques of assessment, monitoring and administration of interventions should ensure that the minimum of pain is suffered in such surgical situations. However, it does seem that in many cases there is substantial moderate to severe pain experienced (Royal Colleges 1990; Paice *et al.* 1991). This can only mean a failure of the service to meet the needs of the patient.

Pain associated with surgery will also include that due to drains, tubes, stitches and their removal. This pain can also be anticipated and prevented. There may also be pain in muscles and joints due to the patient lying in one position for many hours, with heavy instruments lying on top and even doctors and nurses leaning on him or her as they perform the surgery, some of which requires much effort and pushing and pulling. These aches and pains usually recover with rest, but they can make the immediate post-operative period very uncomfortable for the patient.

Fear on anticipation is an important aspect of surgical pain and can be dealt with by information and explanation (Seers 1987; Johnson and Vogele 1993). Often the fear is not about the success of the surgery but about the possibility of pain. There are some forms of surgery associated with changes in lifestyle and ability, such as amputation of a limb, or resection of part of the intestine leading to the creation of a colostomy or similar structure. Anxieties and uncertainties about the future can cloud fear of pain. It is important to sort out the different concerns and deal with them separately and adequately.

Some patients are so relieved to be having treatment (for example, surgery) for their illness (which itself can have been causing great pain and distress) that they do not face the surgery and its associated pain with great fear. Some have reported that the surgical pain was nothing compared with that from their cholecystitis for example (Davis 1984a). Uncertainty about the post-operative experience can be an important factor in the patient's response. This will include what sensations and possible pain to expect, its site and nature, details of resources available. There may also be concern about loss of control of self, of personal functioning, of being dependent on others. Many people have fears and worries about going into hospital and these can be very influential in affecting their response to treatment (Davis 1984b).

Pain from disease (acute)

Although most people have experienced some form of injury pain, probably fewer have experienced pain from disease, excepting perhaps headaches and toothaches.

However, even the common cold or flu can be associated with some degree of pain, such as headaches or more generalised body aches involving muscles and joints. Sometimes the headache can be quite localised and intense. Headaches can occur with symptoms other than those of a cold however, as in migraine, where it is more associated with stress. Here the pain can be much more debilitating as it disturbs the ability to concentrate and think. It can seem to the sufferer to have a particular 'shape' or configuration inside the head which may reflect the route of blood vessels or other structures (see Schoenen *et al.* 1994 for a discussion).

Site

Pain associated with disease is usually located in or near the affected organ or structure. Again it is mainly caused by damage to the tissues involved, or to stretching of, or pressure on, structures. Sometimes the pain can seem to 'run' from one part of the body to another, or to be 'referred' to another (related) part (Procacci *et al.* 1994). This often reflects the way in which the different parts of the body are linked through nerves. Thus if one part of such a section is affected by disease, then the pain may also be experienced in the remaining parts of that section. This can make it difficult sometimes to confirm a diagnosis. The site of the pain as reported by the patient may not seem to make sense in terms of disease. This can happen in appendicitis, or in a case of myocardial infarction, where referred pain is in fact a common diagnostic sign. With appendicitis the pain may be reported from various parts of the abdomen, or even seem to move from one part to another, before settling over the site of the infected appendix. With myocardial infarction, the pain may be reported from the left arm. This experience can be very disconcerting to the patient, adding to the level of anxiety.

The brain, receiving the signals from the periphery, has a limited geography, so to speak, for certain parts. They are not so clearly mapped as others. Areas of high sensitivity (lips, tongue, fingers, eyes, genitalia, feet for example) are given many nerve cells in the brain, as well as having many nerve endings in the actual parts.

Other, relatively insensitive areas have fewer nerve endings and are less well represented in the brain. Thus the sufferer, in attempting to express or describe the pain from these relatively insensitive areas, has less information to go on, and can seem to give a confused or vague picture, and yet in acute situations an accurate diagnosis is important. The person assessing the pain must be aware of this and try to help the patient as much as possible, and try not to get frustrated or to disbelieve him or her.

Some pains associated with disease can be very intense, and cause a shock reaction, so that the person is quite severely incapacitated. For example, that associated with cholecystitis, or with renal colic. Here the pain seems to be caused by muscular spasm as the ducts or ureters involved try to force the respective fluid (bile or urine) past a blockage. Also intense pain can be caused by ischaemia to muscles as in thrombosis in the leg or in the heart for example.

Meaning

When the patient reports pain, therefore, he or she is trying to make sense of signals coming in from various parts of the body. Many different kinds of words can be used by different patients or people in pain to describe their experience (Melzack and Torgerson 1971). With disease there are usually fewer clues as to the cause than with injury. Often the pain is the first indication that there is something wrong. This can be very frightening (and fear or anxiety can increase the likelihood of a shock reaction). The interpretation that the patient puts on the pain will reflect his or her understanding of the body and its processes. There is increasing publicity and information about the body, health and illness in the various media. Many people are now regularly checking their health status. Nevertheless there is often confusion about certain aspects; there may be a tendency to catastrophise the meaning of signals; or a tendency to deny them (see above).

In helping someone to assess their pain, the various meanings that the individual may be attaching to the pain have to be borne in mind in order to come to a realistic interpretation. The person experiencing the pain often has a good idea what it means. Also in this acute situation there is usually some indication that something can be done about it. There can be pain relief in the short term and hopefully a cure or management of the underlying pathology as well. Although some of these pains can signal life-threatening danger, in many cases if diagnosis is efficient then intervention can prevent or reduce the threat to life.

For the sufferer, the intensity and site of the pain can lead to an interpretation of a threat to life. For example, chest pain or abdominal pain seem to be the most feared. The patient will be drawing on memories of others, perhaps family members, who have suffered similar pain. Alternatively they may be aware of lay understandings of the meaning of a particular pain. This will also influence the way in which they express or report the pain.

Pain from disease (chronic)

Sometimes pain from an acute disease situation can fail to be cured and enter into a long-term or chronic state. This is usually defined as pain that continues for more than three months. Pain from bones, joints and the lower back in particular are common types under this heading. It can be associated with an injury as perhaps in some low back pain, or in some cases of low back pain there may be no obvious damage (CSAG 1994). There may be general wear and tear linked with disease as in arthritic or rheumatic conditions. There may be disease of the nervous system itself causing chronic pain, and some headaches can be chronic (Schoenen *et al.* 1994). Neurogenic pain is associated with damage or disease of the nervous system and this can lead to a very severe burning kind of pain which is very difficult to treat. Types include causalgia, various neuralgias, and even phantom pain, although this latter is still a great mystery (Melzack and Wall 1996).

Meaning

The management of chronic pain often presents the greatest challenge to the health-care professionals. This is where the individual interpretation and meaning given to the pain by the sufferer can influence greatly the ability to cope with or to reduce the pain. If the chronic pain is also seen as ultimately a signal of a life-threatening condition as in cancer, then this also affects the meaning of and response to the pain (Roy 1992). Most chronic pain does not augur a life threatening situation, merely a life-reducing or -limiting situation. It is the impact on the sufferer's quality of life that is often the main issue to be addressed.

Sometimes there are successful regimes that can help to reduce the severity of pain so that the patient is able to carry on a normal life. However, there are many situations where treatment is not so effective and other measures have to be introduced which deal with the psycho-social aspects of the pain experience (see Roy 1992 for a discussion of these aspects). Helping the sufferer to interpret the pain in such a way that they can cope more effectively with the pain, or to help the interventions being provided to be more effective, is the challenge. Getting the inside story of the pain so that there is a better understanding of the patient's experience is the problem facing the caring professional. It is important to try to understand the particular factors that are operating and influencing the way the sufferer gives meaning to the pain and thus is affected by it.

Emotions

Feelings of helplessness are not uncommon, and may be associated with a depressive reaction. Alternatively there may be feelings of self-blame for misdeeds in the past for which the pain is a punishment. Some people have a strong religious bent and may interpret the pain as a challenge from God or a punishment from God. The pain may inspire feelings of regret for steps taken in the past; feelings that 'if only', things would not be as they are now (Walker *et al.* 1990).

Lifestyle

The person suffering from chronic pain has to face the prospect of long-term changes to their lifestyle, which may become very limited. This limitation may very well affect their partners or family who will also be influencing the sufferer's reaction to the pain. These psycho-social factors and also cultural factors may be very powerful indeed and treatments or interventions will be viewed through these influences.

There may well be economic consequences to the chronic pain, in terms of lost or reduced opportunities to work. Issues of compensation and litigation may compound the issue (Skevington 1995; Melzack and Wall 1996). The sense of self-worth associated with being a productive independent person will be affected. Self-esteem or lack of it can be very influential in determining an individual's reaction to chronic pain. Ability or desire to cope constructively with the pain may be reduced if a sense of low esteem, depression, loss of control of one's life are operating. These reactions can influence the efficacy of interventions that otherwise might work. Thus the professional, particularly the nurse, has a most important role to play in helping the sufferer gain a more positive interpretation of the situation, to give the pain a different meaning so that they can be encouraged and enabled to allow relevant interventions to work at their maximum.

Life-threatening situations

If there is a life-threatening or a terminal situation developing then the psycho-social aspects can become increasingly delicate as can the pharmacological one. Dying in a pain-free and dignified way is an expectation and hope we all have. To be approaching, consciously and slowly, one's end, in pain and distress, puts great demands on the individual, physically, emotionally and spiritually (Penson and Fisher 1991). No one can ever really know what it is like for another at such a time. And yet if we are to contribute meaningfully and constructively to someone's pain-free and dignified death the more insight that we can gain into the possible factors and processes that might be operating the better. The nature of our relationship with the dying person, whereby we demonstrate a desire to share with them their 'inside story', will be crucial. They and they alone should be the arbiters of their care.

Unusual pain situations

As we have emphasised it is most important to get the patient's views on the nature, severity and site of pain, as well as their evaluation of the effectiveness of any treatment. It is an extra challenge when we come across people who might be in pain but who have difficulty in communicating that pain to us, certainly in a form of communication that we can understand. If it is a question of language difficulty then the use of interpreters can be invaluable. Alternatively, non-verbal systems can be utilised, using sign language perhaps.

However, if the patient does not have the level of intellectual development to be able to communicate in a meaningful way, through some learning difficulty or through extreme youth, such as the pre-verbal infant, particularly the neonatal infant, then special circumstances apply.

Learning disabilities

With people with learning disabilities it may be possible to gain some information through sign language or observations of behaviours, when at least the site of the pain might be revealed. This will involve non-verbal communication and the ability to assess and interpret cues of all kinds. The sufferer in this situation may not even have the ability to think about their pain in other than simple, non-verbal concepts of unpleasantness, or avoidance. There will be an inability to explain the pain resulting from injury for example, depending on the degree of disability. The nature of the relationship developed between such a person and their carers will be vitally important in trying to gain some insight as to what they are experiencing. The observer must be looking for other signs of injury or disease which might indicate the presence of pain. Disturbed behaviour which might represent the frustration and agony that otherwise cannot be expressed must be studied for this possible interpretation.

The elderly

In an ageing person with such difficulties of communication, there must be an expectation that there might be pain from, say, arthritis, or from other degenerative disorders. Postural changes, guarding of parts of the body, or rubbing or massaging painful parts might give clues. Caring for people with such problems demands the highest level of professional skill, knowledge and sensitivity (Walker *et al.* 1990). There are also many psychological factors operating with the elderly, related to their past experience, which must be assessed, discussed and catered for.

Infants and neonates

Very young infants have similar problems of inability to communicate. Often, if born prematurely, or with some health problem occurring soon after birth, there is the need to perform painful interventions and surgery. Even pre-term infants have nervous systems developed in order to sense and experience pain (e.g. Anand and Hickey 1987; Torres and Anderson 1985). There is no doubt that these very young infants have some experience which echoes the adult experience of pain. There is not the language or experience or learning to help to explain or give meaning to the experience.

Nevertheless it is still very unpleasant, can cause a strong shock reaction, behavioural disturbances, and is totally unnecessary. If pain would have been caused by an intervention, medical or surgical, in an adult or older child then it must be assumed that an equally unpleasant sensation is being experienced by the infant. All attempts must be made to prevent or treat it.

Generally we assume that being born and coming into contact with light, noise and touch in the outside environment is not too pleasant. We usually go to great lengths to comfort, and calm, newborn infants. We keep them warm and quiet and comforted with food (milk), stroking and cuddling them.

Tied to a splint and with needles and tubes entering all orifices, with cuts through the skin to provide access to veins for cannulae for infusions, life is not pleasant for the neonatal infant requiring intensive care. And yet it is not unusual for no analgesic to be given (Mather and Mackie 1983; Beyer and Byers 1985), not even anaesthetic skin cream to ease injections. Non-verbal clues and common sense can help to appreciate what is being experienced and thus to try to alleviate any pain or distress. Again this kind of care demands a very high level of professional expertise and sensitivity.

Not feeling any pain

In some rare situations it has been reported that under great stress and with other demands on them some individuals have undergone severe trauma and yet have not reported pain, or, seemingly, been aware of any (Melzack *et al.* 1982). There are other individuals who seem to be able to control their pain reactions and to undergo what would otherwise be very painful experiences such as burning or piercing with hooks. Yet others seem not to have been born with the ability to feel pain, or much other sensation. These people are thus very vulnerable to injury, without pain as a signal of danger (Scadding 1994). The existence of such reactions or non-reaction to pain is still very much a puzzle and tells us that there is still very much more to learn and understand about the phenomenon (Melzack and Wall 1996).

Phantom pain

There are also those who feel pain when there seems to be no longer anything to feel pain, as in amputation of a limb. This situation offers a great challenge to the health-care professional (Merskey 1986). The pain seems very real to the sufferer yet there is nothing there to treat. Although the body has lost a part, the brain still has the old geography, so to speak, wired in, and presumably sees no reason why there should not still be pain coming from that part, if the signals coming in suggest that it might be. Also changes have been identified in the central nervous system as a result of injury or surgical section (Wall and Jones 1991). Such pain can seem very intense to the sufferer. This is another mystery area and one which, if we can gain more insight into it, might tell us more about the whole process of the experience of pain, and how it might be managed.

Conclusion

From the picture described above then it will be seen that pain is a very complex phenomenon. It involves a wide range of academic disciplines as well as professional areas. There is much research evidence now accumulated around the area. The point of this chapter has been to try to demonstrate the essential variety of the pain experience, depending on the nature of the pain situation, and the variety of ways in which that experience can be interpreted depending on who is doing the interpreting.

We are never dealing with Mr or Mrs Average. There are no standard reactions to a pain-producing experience. There may be certain principles that can be applied as we attempt to identify individual needs in people suffering from pain and as we attempt to help them gain relief. Indeed there can be tendencies to react in a particular way, as demonstrated by a qualitative study involving interviews with chronic pain patients (Carson and Mitchell 1998). Three themes were identified from the analysis. The first indicated that patients felt that the pain wore them down, but that they felt that they should get on with it and make do. The second theme dealt with the tendency to tell and yet also not to tell about the pain experience. The patients tended to reveal themselves differently to different people. The third theme was about the role that hope for relief plays in enabling the sufferers to carry on.

Nevertheless, at the end of the day we must remember that the pain is the patient's. Only he or she experiences it and gives it meaning. We are very much on the outside trying to get in. It is a multi-disciplinary and multi-professional job to gain the 'inside story', but gain it we must if we are really to care for people in pain.

The experience of pain can be divided into four aspects (Melzack and Wall 1996). These are, the sensory-discriminative; the emotional-motivational; the cognitive-evaluative; and the social and cultural aspects. In the following four chapters we shall deal with each of these, reviewing evidence to gain an understanding of the experience of pain by individuals. From these separate aspects we shall then be in a better position to appreciate the holistic experience and thus form a better approach to the assessment and management of that pain experience.

Part II

Factors influencing the pain experience

Chapter 3

Nociception

Sensory-discriminative aspects

> Pleasure is a visitant, but
> Pain clings cruelly to us
> Keats

Introduction

Although we have argued that pain can be seen as 'all in the mind', as an interpretation, a meaning given to neuronal activity in the brain, it does seem on the whole to originate in signals received from the periphery. Nerve endings in the skin and other organs send signals along sensory fibres to the central nervous system, usually via the spinal cord whence the information is transmitted to the brain and central processing. It is there that these signals are combined with others from other centres in the brain or from other parts of the body and are then interpreted as pain.

In this chapter we shall be concentrating on the flow of information through the nervous system from those nerve endings to the centres in the brain. It is important to remember that the system acts as a whole, and that other cognitive and emotional centres in the brain are an integral part of the pain experience. Also it is important to remember that not all pain experienced has an obvious source at the periphery. Nevertheless it is useful to study the parts separately in order to more fully understand the whole process. Unusual situations can then be considered, but following the same principles.

In many ways we need to leap-frog from nociceptive, to cognitive-emotional, to socio-cultural aspects all at once to see the process in action. This is not possible without a great deal of confusion. Therefore it would seem better to proceed more slowly and in sections before we put the whole process together when we look at ways of helping the person in pain. Then these sections can more easily and perhaps more meaningfully come together. We shall start with the periphery at the nerve endings and follow the stimulus towards the spinal cord and from there further into the central nervous system and the various parts of the brain that are involved in creating the particular experience of pain that a sufferer might have. Before that however it is important that we consider the main approaches to the understanding of pain and attempts to explain the pain mechanism and experience. Three main theories are generally considered to have been influential. They are the Specificity Theory, the Pattern Theory and the Gate Control Theory.

Theories of pain

Specificity Theory

The principle behind this approach is that there are specific nerves and nerve endings that send signals to specific pain centres in the brain so that pain can be experienced. This theory has had a long life, and was clearly described in the seventeenth century by the philosopher Descartes (see Melzack and Wall (1996) for a critical review of these theories). However, although it does seem attractive and there is some evidence as to how nerves and parts of the central nervous system work which might support it, there is also strong evidence that offers the alternative view, that it is not an adequate explanation. For example, the theory does acknowledge the role of thin A-delta fibres and C fibres in the nociceptive process, and also the spino-thalamic tracts as playing a part in the transmission of signals to the brain. However, there is much evidence to show that there is not necessarily a direct link between site of injury and experience of pain by the individual, for example evidence from surgery on nerves, or the experience of phantom limb pain. Some people do not experience pain although there might be an obvious injury (Beecher 1959). Similarly the different meanings given to similar types of pain situation (e.g. injury, chronic or cancer pain) by different people argues strongly for other mechanisms to be interacting with the nociceptive system (Melzack and Wall 1996). It seems that there is some degree of specificity in the peripheral nervous system. Further discussion of this point is given below when we look at the activity of the neurones in more detail.

Pattern Theory

An alternative approach to the Specificity Theory suggested that it was the pattern of signals that identified a particular set of signals as being 'pain' signals. Thus there was a summation of information at say the dorsal horn of the spinal cord where a particular spatial or temporal patterning could be identified. This originated with the work of Goldscheider in the last century (1894; see Melzack and Wall 1996), but has since been developed and argued by more recent theorists such as Noordenbos (1959) and Weddell (1955). This model is in contrast to the straight through model of specificity. The possibility that there might be stages in the progress of the signals where decisions were made as to the nature of the signal, and involving different fibres synapsing with each other in the spinal cord, helped in some way to overcome some of the criticisms of specificity. It has also helped to lay the ground for the development of the theory that at present seems to be able to explain and predict many of the phenomena associated with the experience of pain.

Gate Control Theory

Gate Control Theory was originally proposed by Melzack and Wall (1965). The original proposal showed the connections at the dorsal horn level (see Figure 3.1). The proposal was that thin nociceptive A-delta and C fibres synapsed with the large A-beta fibres, in the substantia gelatinosa (SG). The A-beta fibres have an inhibiting effect on the signals from the thin fibres at relatively low levels of intensity. The A-delta and C fibres also synapse with transmission (T) cells which themselves synapse with ascending fibres to the brain and action systems. If not inhibited by the A-beta fibres then the signals travel via the T cells to the higher centres for interpretation and action. This inhibiting effect produced a kind of gating mechanism where the A-beta fibres could close the gate and prevent or reduce the nociceptive stimulus.

Melzack and Wall (1996) argue that any new theory must be able to explain the following phenomena: the highly variable relationship between injury and pain; pain may be produced by apparently innocuous stimuli; the location of pain may not correlate with the location of damage; pain may continue when healing has occurred or may exist when there is no injury; the nature and location of pain

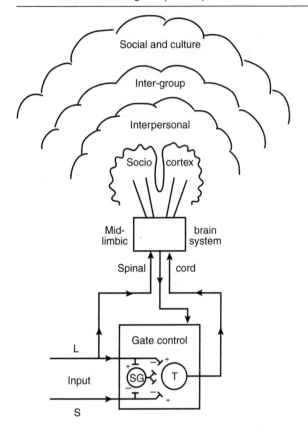

Figure 3.1   Socio-cultural extension of the gate control model of pain

Source: after Melzack and Wall (1996) and Skevington (1995); previously
published in B. Carter (ed.) (1998) *Perspectives on Pain: Mapping the
Territory*, London: Arnold

Notes: L   large diameter fibres; S   small diameter fibres; SG   substantia
gelatinosa; T   transmission cells; +   excitation; −   inhibition

may change over time; pain has many dimensions; and some types
of pain cannot be treated. In the following sections of this chapter
we shall explore the sensory-discriminative aspects of the pain experience, demonstrating the gate control system in action so to speak.
In the following three chapters we shall then explore the emotional-
motivational, cognitive-evaluative, and social and cultural aspects.

Neuronal activity

The following descriptions of the relevant parts of the nervous system are in a relatively summary form. More detail should be sought from specialised textbooks of neuro-anatomy.

Nerve endings

In the sensory nervous system, signals start at receptors. These are the ends of the axons which branch out from the cell body of the neurone (see Figure 3.2). Many of these are highly specialised, such as those for sight, hearing, taste and smell. These are also associated with specific sense organs where the nerve endings are sited. There are other senses however which are not so localised. Balance, for example, and sense of what position our body is in are associated with special nerve endings in muscles, joints and the inner ear. The sensation of fullness after a meal is based on signals from receptors in the stomach and intestines.

Among the general sensory nerve endings there seems to be some differentiation in function. There does seem to be a sensitivity to light touch which might give rise to the sensation of tickle or being stroked or caressed. Also there is a sensitivity to heavy pressure. Finally there seems to be a sensitivity to temperature change or chemicals, including those released by damaged tissue (Meyer *et al.* 1994). There have been attempts to identify specialised nerve endings and some do seem to have a specific structure. However, such

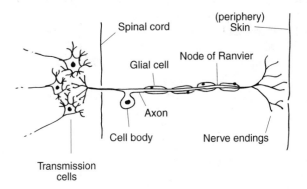

Figure 3.2   Sensory neurone indicating the link between the periphery and the spinal cord

specialised nerve endings do not appear at all sites in the periphery and their exact purpose is not really clear (Melzack and Wall 1996).

Neurones

Not only are the receptors or nerve endings sensitive to different stimuli, but the actual nerve fibres themselves vary in size of diameter (thick or thin) and as to whether or not they are covered by a myelin sheath made of Glial cells. These are the axons extending from the cell bodies to the next neurones where they meet their dendrites and form synapses. These differences in size influence the rate at which impulses travel along the fibres. Thus we have fast, 30–100 msec., thick and myelinated fibres (A-beta fibres); slow, 6–30 msec., thin and myelinated fibres (A-delta fibres); and very slow, 1–2.5 msec., thin and unmyelinated fibres (C fibres) (Melzack and Wall 1996; Bentley 1998). The myelin sheath speeds up the process of transmission of the electrical signal along the fibres by acting as an insulation sheath.

There does seem to be some specialisation of function among the neurones, regarding pain. The A-delta and C fibres seem to be the main nociceptors. The large, myelinated A-beta fibres are associated with light pressure, and have the ability to block A-delta and C fibres when there is a low-intensity signal. The thin, myelinated A-delta fibres are associated with light pressure, heavy pressure, chemicals and temperature change (heating or cooling). The thin, unmyelinated C fibres are associated with light pressure, heavy pressure, chemicals and temperature change (heating). Two-thirds of all sensory fibres are of the thin, unmyelinated C type. They may be polymodal in that each may respond to different types of stimulus. Some of the thin, myelinated A-delta fibres are also polymodal. Some of these differences in modality are related to firing rates of the neurone – the frequency at which the impulses pass along the fibre (Melzack and Wall 1996).

The inflammatory response

The inflammatory response, such as that occurring with a sprain, when tissues are stretched or torn, provides a good example of the chemical stimulation of nerve endings to produce pain. When the C fibres sense the chemicals released by the damaged tissue, 5 hydroxytryptamine, the bradykinins, histamine and the prostaglandins, for example, then peptides such as substance P, and neurokinins A and B, are produced by the C fibres (the axon effect) which then stimulate the nociceptive signal to the centre (Rang and Bevan 1994). The sympathetic nerves release noradrenaline, acetylcholine and adenosine, adding to the effect. Thus is achieved the perception and continuation of the feeling of pain from the sprain. An important part of this process is played by arachidonic acid, which, under the influence of the cyclo-oxygenases 1 and 2, produces prostaglandins which are an important part of the inflammatory process too. Certain drugs interfere with the action of the cyclo-oxygenases (the non-steroidal anti-inflammatory drugs, NSAIDs), which we shall consider in Chapter 7.

Thus we can see that a wide variety of information may be transmitted at varying rates to the central nervous system (CNS), with the combination of different sensitivities at the receptors, and the different types of nerve fibre.

Synapses

There is not, of course, one long fibre from the nerve ending in the skin, say, to the brain. There is a series of fibres linked by synapses, where information is transmitted from fibre to fibre. A fibre from the skin, for example, will travel to the spinal cord where it will synapse with a fibre in the spinal cord. Within the spinal cord there are many synapses between fibres. These include those between sensory fibres from the periphery and internal fibres communicating with other parts of the spinal cord (short ones) and those communicating with the brain and higher centres (long ones). There are also direct synapses with motor fibres to produce reflex responses to certain types of stimulation.

At the synapse, chemicals are released by the incoming fibre which are then received by the next fibre and these then stimulate the electrical signal in the second fibre which then transmits the signal to its other end where a similar chemical transmission will occur at the next synapse (see Figure 3.3). Many chemical transmitters have been identified, such as acetylcholine, dopamine, serotonin, and substance P. They may have either a stimulating or inhibiting function depending on the nature of the synapse. This ability to either continue the transmission of the signal or to inhibit it offers an important opportunity to influence or modify the signal and thus the kind of message that is received in the higher centres.

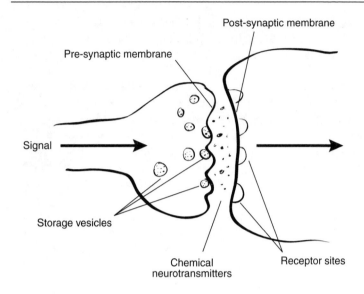

Figure 3.3   A synapse. The junction may be between dendrites and
dendrites; dendrites and axons; axons and axons or other
multiple combinations

In the central nervous system, and in particular in the brain, the
various functions are achieved by these links between many different
fibres from different sources and centres. Our ability to perceive
light, sound, taste, touch and pain and to give it meaning is the
result of many such links between millions of nerve cells sharing
information in the form of electrical signals mediated through
chemical transmitters at the synapses. We shall discuss further the
actions of the chemical transmitters when we consider the functions
of these higher centres.

Spinal cord

The spinal cord has a particular structure to facilitate the transmission of signals up towards the brain and more central parts of the
CNS, and down from these central parts to the periphery. However,
there are also neurones which merely communicate between other
neurones within the spinal cord. The sensory neurones from the
periphery enter the spinal cord in particular areas, in the dorsal
horn of the central grey matter where clusters of nerves are grouped

into plexuses serving a particular part of the body. For example, we have the cervical plexus which consists of neurones entering the lower cervical cord and the upper thoracic cord. These neurones from the arm and the upper chest are linked in the spinal cord and reflect the outgrowth of the arm from the thoracic area in the embryo. The nerves from the leg and the pelvis are similarly linked in the lumbosacral plexus. The relatively few neurones from the abdominal and lower thoracic periphery are not so strongly linked or co-ordinated. However, there is a strong plexus associated with the diaphragmatic and epigastric regions internally, the solar plexus. This helps to explain some of the apparently strange experiences of moving pains or referred pains.

Following the track of signals coming into the central nervous system from the periphery, then the synapse occurs in the dorsal horn of the grey matter (consisting mainly of the cell bodies of the neurones) (see Figure 3.4). The dorsal horn comprises layers or laminae of cells extending from the surface to the central area around the cerebro-spinal canal. The A-delta and C fibres enter laminae i and ii; A-beta fibres enter laminae iii and iv. Finally a mixture of A-beta and A-delta enter lamina v. Links between the laminae are achieved and maintained through chemical neurotrans-mitters (Melzack and Wall 1996). Laminae i and ii are dark and visible to the naked eye because they consist largely of the cell bodies, and are known as the substantia gelatinosa.

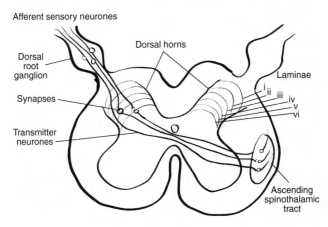

Figure 3.4   Diagram of a section of the spinal cord indicating the dorsal horns and the sensory signal route to the ascending spinothalamic tract via the dorsal horn laminae

It is in the laminae i and ii that Melzack and Wall (1965) assumed that the gate control mechanism operates. However, more recently they propose that the gate control phenomenon is more complex and should incorporate the ascending and descending systems as well (Melzack and Wall 1996). This will be discussed in more detail below when the descending system is described.

The neurones linking the dorsal horn with the rest of the central nervous system have axons that ascend the spinal cord along various tracts and to various parts of the brain, such as the reticular formation, the limbic system and the thalamus. The reticular formation seems to have a co-ordinating function (Yaksh 1986).

The brain

In essence in the brain, the signal reaches the sensory cortex from whence it can be distributed to other centres in the brain for further analysis and the attribution of meaning, linking with emotions and motor activity. In the sensory cortex the different parts of the body are given their own section so to speak so that a representation of the body is created reflecting the relative importance, in terms of sensation, of the various parts of the body.

However, before it reaches the sensory cortex the signal synapses with neurones in other centres in the medulla and midbrain. These play an important part in the meaning attributed to the pain experience. They define the kind of experience the person will have, at an emotional, motivational level. Also this part plays a major role in the gate control mechanism.

Reticular formation

At the top of the spinal cord the signals from the periphery arrive at the medulla. This forms an important part of a network of centres (the reticular net-like formation) including the midbrain, sensory thalamus and hypothalamus. The nucleus gigantocellularis of the medulla seems to be a centre for strong aversive (avoidance) responses to sensory inputs (Casey et al. 1974). The central grey area of the midbrain similarly produces a strong aversive response.

The reticular formation seems to have a central, integrating function in the pain experience. It has been shown that neurones in these centres also link with other centres, such as those in the limbic system (Casey 1980).

Limbic system

This links with the reticular formation via the central grey area of the midbrain. The limbic system comprises the hippocampus, the amygdala, and the cingulate gyrus among other centres. They link with the medial thalamus and the hypothalamus to the frontal cortex. The limbic system can be seen as one of the main emotion centres of the brain (Bouckoms 1994).

Here we get approach responses as well as avoidance ones, particularly in the hypothalamus. Some centres can vary their response from approach at low stimulation to avoidance at high levels of stimulation. There is evidence that cognitive maps are built up in these centres (O'Keefe and Nadel 1978), particularly the hippocampus and the amygdala which link spatial relationships associated with the incoming stimuli in the hippocampus, with positive or negative affective (emotional) information associated with past experiences in the amygdala (Gloor 1978). There is also evidence that the perceived size of the site of the pain changes with changes in the level of attention paid to it (P. A. McGrath 1990).

Links with the ventrobasal part of the thalamus and the somatosensory cortex then allow information about the precise location of the stimulation at the periphery to be included in the experience. Once the cortex has been included then there is access to information from all other sensory inputs, including the special senses which can become part of the experience and the particular meaning and memory of the pain experience. There is also access to previous meaning and memory information to add to the experience. The location of the pain experience, therefore, would seem to be established in the ventrobasal thalamus and the sensory cortex through links with other centres in the brain (Melzack and Wall 1996).

We can thus see that a large variety of patterns of information can reach the higher centres in the brain, and thus awareness, to create the experience of pain. We have a sensory-discriminative pattern; a motivation-affective pattern; and cognitive-evaluative pattern. The variety of nerve endings, the different types of nerve fibre and the various links with different centres on the way to the centre, all serve to produce very different types of experience. Recent research has attempted to demonstrate these links (sensory-discriminative and cognitive-evaluative using MRI and PET scans, with some success (Treede *et al.* 1999; Jones 1997)).

However, it seems that the communication is not all one way.

One of the most important insights into the pain experience has been that of the understanding that there are descending signals which affect the incoming ascending signals before they reach the sensory cortex, and awareness and appreciation of the experience of pain. It is also possible for activity at a cortical cognitive level to influence ongoing incoming pain signals, so that the pain experience may be modified, and to a certain extent controlled.

Descending system

As indicated above, the A-beta fibres also synapse with ascending neurones which project up to the higher centres (including the medulla, midbrain and thalamus) and thus help to stimulate the descending system which can also inhibit (or stimulate) the A-delta and C fibres. Further exploration of the functions of the reticular formation (medulla, midbrain, thalamus), in particular the periaqueductal grey matter, has shown that certain substances are produced which have an analgesic effect, the opioids enkephalins, dynorphins or endorphins, first discovered by Hughes *et al.* (1975). They are produced in the pituitary gland, and appear throughout the brain and spinal cord (Fields and Basbaum 1994; Woolf and Wall 1983). They are neuropeptides and act as inhibiting neurotransmitters. Their production is stimulated by other chemical mediators, such as serotonin.

Fibres from the cerebral cortex, cerebellum and from the hypothalamus are received by the periaqueductal grey matter which is rich in enkephalins and opiate receptors. From there other fibres connect with the nucleus raphe magnus and the nucleus reticularis gigantocellularis in the medulla which are rich in serotonin, from whence other fibres descend to the dorsal horn of the spinal cord via the dorsolateral funiculus (see Figure 3.5). Here they enter the laminae of the horn and produce inhibition of signals coming in from the periphery by affecting the transmission neurones (Fields and Basbaum 1994). This is achieved by the secretion of serotonin and noradrenaline to stimulate the release of the endorphins, dynorphins and enkephalins (Basbaum and Fields 1978). This enhances the gating mechanism. Thus the gating mechanism is seen as applying to this whole process, involving the dorsal horn, the higher centres and the ascending and descending tracts, as one system (Melzack and Wall 1996).

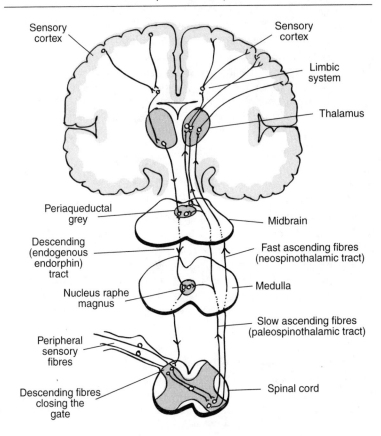

Figure 3.5   The ascending and descending pain pathways

Pain in children and infants

As indicated in the first chapter there is evidence of under-medication of young children and particularly of neonates in the management of pain. There are many myths and misconceptions about the pain experience in infants and young children, as have been described thoroughly by McCaffrey *et al.* (1994). They include the almost general doubt that infants and young children really can feel pain or need analgesics; also there is the misconception that a denial of pain means no pain (many children fear the intervention to relieve pain more than the pain). Similarly a failure to report pain does not mean no pain, the child and even the parent of the child in pain may not realise that they must tell the professionals that there is pain. The ability to distract the child from the pain does not mean it is not severe. Certainly children are no more able to tolerate pain than are adults, many versions of opiate drugs are now available and it is relatively safe to administer them, provided the usual precautions are taken against side effects or toxic effects (see Chapter 7). There is no evidence that young children are likely to become addicted either.

The mechanism of pain as described in this chapter occurs in neonates as well as infants and young children. There is evidence that young children and neonates have the neuronal links to have cognitive awareness of a painful stimulus. Although myelination is not fully achieved at birth it progresses very rapidly and, even then, does not seem to be essential for the transmission of nerve impulses to the cortex. This applies also to adults (Price and Dubner 1977). The foetus has sensory innervation to all subcutaneous areas and the cortex has its full complement of neurones by the 20th week of gestation (Vaughan 1975; Anand and Hickey 1987). Evoked cortical activity has been identified in response to auditory, olfactory and tactile stimuli (Torres and Anderson 1985), and endorphins have been identified in the amniotic fluid in relation to foetal distress (Gautrey et al. 1977).

Behavioural responses demonstrate that there is distress as a result of particular experiences that in adults would cause pain. These include body movement (Craig et al. 1984; Franck 1986); facial expression (the pain face) (Johnston and Strada 1986; Grunau and Craig 1987) (see Figure 9.4 in Chapter 9 on assessment of pain in children). Also cries have been used to identify pain in infants (Wolff 1974; Levine and Gordon 1982). Certain aspects of physiological activity have also been shown to change in the pain situation, indicating at least a stress reaction, for example, heart rate increase (Beaver 1987), blood pressure (Beaver 1987; Brown 1987), and endocrine changes such as noradrenaline and blood glucose increases (Anand et al. 1985).

It is most important therefore that those looking after young children and infants are aware of the facts and do not allow the myths and misconceptions about pain to interfere with good, individualised management of the pain.

Conclusion

The person experiencing pain, therefore, is sitting on the top of a hierarchy of inter-related neurones so to speak, which are transmitting signals both up and down the central nervous system. From this plethora of signals, some from different centres in the brain and some almost directly from the periphery, involving sensory-discriminative, emotional and motivational, cognitive-evaluative, and action information, a meaning is created and the pain experienced.

The person, the aware self, thus experiences a pain that reflects the kind of stimulation at the periphery; the nature of the neurones communicating that sensation to the spinal cord; the nature of the kinds of links made with neurones in the spinal cord; the nature of links made with higher centres in the brain, such as the medulla, midbrain and thalamus; the nature of any links made with cortical centres including the somatosensory centre, but including others which enable memory, and social and cultural influences, to play a part.

The nature of a particular pain experience is dependent on the particular mixture of influences at each of the possible junctions in the route from periphery to centre. The pain experience is therefore essentially subjective and individual and 'all in the mind', with its own 'inside story' or pattern of influences along the route. The person calls this experience 'pain'. Only the sufferer knows when it is, where it is and what it feels like.

This chapter has largely been about the sensory-discriminative aspect of the pain experience. In the following chapters we shall concentrate on the emotional-motivational, cognitive-evaluative and socio-cultural aspects. Whereas the sensory-discriminative aspect has been demonstrated from the viewpoint of neuro-anatomy, the other aspects will be demonstrated from the viewpoint of psychology and sociology.

Chapter 4

Emotional and motivational aspects of pain

A man who fears suffering is already suffering from what he fears.
Michel de Montaigne

Introduction

There is always an emotional aspect to a pain experience. There is also always some level of drive to respond. The person having the experience will be aware of emotions generated by the experience. The common feelings are fear and anxiety and depression. However, other feelings are experienced depending on the person and the situation, such as feelings of guilt, pride (in coping), anger (why me?), helplessness, or loneliness. However, emotions also play a most important role in our lives outside of the pain experience. Many people feel that they are what life is all about. Looking at the worlds of poetry, literature and art we find that they are the mainsprings of quality of life.

Feelings, emotions, are most important for satisfactorily dealing with life events. They can be seen as being grounded in avoidance and approach reactions which, as we have seen in the previous chapter, are an essential part of the experience of pain (Casey *et al.* 1974). Centres in the brain, the reticular formation and the limbic system in particular, have important links with the sympathetic and parasympathetic nervous systems as well as the cortical areas of the brain. From the basic approach and avoidance responses, generated in these centres, and in particular the hypothalamus, which is a major component, the various visceral and cognitive elaborations of the emotions can then be experienced (Casey 1980). The emotions are also closely linked with the action centres, mainly motor driven, whereby we can express them (Treede *et al.* 1999). An inability to act on emotions, leading to frustration and a sense of helplessness, can be important concomitants of emotional responses, either approach or, in the case of pain, avoidance.

The nature of the emotional reaction will vary according to the nature of the pain situation. A range of types of pain situation were discussed in Chapter 2 (e.g. P. A. McGrath 1990; Turk and Melzack 1992), and the emotions associated with the various kinds will differ accordingly. Anxiety would seem to be more strongly associated with acute pain and with anticipated pain. It is often the uncertainty of anticipation that provokes the anxiety. Depression is more strongly associated with chronic pain situations, particularly when associated with incurable disease as in cancer or with approaching death in terminal illness. There may be also anxiety in the latter situation. Depression can also be associated with anger and a sense of helplessness. There may be a sense of guilt or of being punished for some behaviour in the past. Not infrequently, with the elderly, chronic pain may be associated with a sense of regret over decisions made in the past (Walker *et al.* 1990).

Thus the person receiving signals from the periphery (where ever that might be, or seem to be) will have associated with them emotional reactions, based on the avoidance/approach reactions in the reticular formation and the limbic system. The nature of the emotional reaction, elaborated by past experience and other cognitive processes, will colour the interpretation of the signals and thus the meaning given to them, i.e. pain of a particular type.

In exploring with the person in pain their experience in order to care for them, the emotional aspects can offer most valuable information for developing interventions and coping strategies to suit that particular person. Nurses are in a very good position to play a therapeutic role in this area. Many interventions are available to help the person in pain to face their emotional reactions, which offer techniques to help the person to move towards more positive emotional responses, and thus to a stronger coping state. The link between the physical and the cognitive is very important here also and will be addressed in some detail in a later chapter.

In the following section we shall look at the nature of emotional reactions in general and in particular with regard to pain. As emotions affect the drive or motivation to want to do something about the situation, then we shall consider that aspect in the final section.

Emotional aspects of pain

When we come to look at the emotional aspects of pain we can draw on our understanding of the emotions in general to help us to support the person experiencing the pain and their particular emotions. Although we have identified a range of emotions which human beings can experience, in the following sections we shall be concentrating on anxiety and stress, and depression, as those that seem to be most frequently reported. However, we shall mention others in passing.

Fear, anxiety and stress

Fear, anxiety and stress are related but slightly different phenomena. Fear is obviously an anticipation of an event, but often with an unknown outcome. Information from the periphery, including the eyes and ears, as well as our memory and thinking processes can stimulate a feeling of fear. The feeling becomes anxiety when focused on a particular event or situation, such as an examination or a visit to the dentist, or an operation. However, some people do experience what is known as 'free floating' anxiety, which does not seem to have a focus. Stress is a word that refers to the stimulus and to the response. The use of the word stressor as the threat or stimulus helps to clarify things, with the word stress as the response (Lazarus and Folkman 1984).

Cannon and Baird (1929 and 1934 respectively) first identified the psychological and physical links embodying anxiety. They argued that this response created three alternative reactions: fright, flight or fight. There are both physical and mental stimuli operating, and they proposed that the same physical visceral responses operated for all emotions. This has been disputed (see Ekman 1992; Levenson 1992). The subjective experiences do seem to differ between individuals (Larsen and Diener 1987).

Weiner (1985) developed the idea of attributions of meanings to events, and proposed that they were of the order good–bad, or pleasant–unpleasant, and related to internal or external factors. This latter relates to the earlier work of Rotter (1966) and his theory of internal and external locus of control. From this it is postulated that those with a tendency to seek explanations or a sense of responsibility within themselves tend to experience less anxiety. Those with a tendency to find explanations dependent on other people or outside agencies tend to experience more anxiety (Beck *et al.* 1985). This idea of the individual evaluating the threat and responding in the light of that evaluation was further developed by Lazarus (1980) and Lazarus and Folkman (1984). They postulated from their research that the appraisal of the threat by the individual, and its meaning in the light of the physiological and cognitive reaction, leads to a particular coping reaction and the identification of a particular emotion. Ekman and Friesen (1969) and Ekman *et al.* (1983) have argued that the meaning of an emotional experience may be created by a behavioural response, such as grinning and bearing it. They argued that certain facial expressions are innate and that the facial expression can stimulate the emotion.

The stressor can produce a positive response as the individual accepts the challenge of the stimulus and seeks ways of coping with the threat. However, there can also be a negative response if there is no way of relieving the uncertainty that causes the situation and the stress becomes anxiety rather than a challenge. This interpersonal or individual aspect of stress responses is the main focus of Lazarus and Folkman's transactional process theory of stress (1984). Each individual makes an appraisal of the situation and determines for him or herself the nature of threat, if any, contained within it. Spielberger (1966) also uses the same principle for his approach to anxiety, as does Mishel (1988) for his approach to uncertainty. The anxiety and the uncertainty is entirely as perceived by the individual. Some might find a situation exciting, others might find it frightening, and yet others find it anxiety provoking.

The experience of anxiety and fear

Some people get a sense of thrill from putting themselves in a fear-provoking situation, but one in which there are safeguards against anything actually happening. Thus frightening and horrifying films can be 'enjoyed' from the safety of a cinema seat, or one's own sitting room. Similarly some sport and other recreational activities can offer the thrill of fear as part of their attraction. However, real fear, of an event over which one has little or no control, is a rather different thing. Here there is a physiological reaction and a mental response that is far more acute than anything offered in the cinema or sport. In many ways one would expect feelings of fear and anxiety to be experienced prior to surgery for example or before a visit to the dentist. Most people will have experienced the latter, and it will occur however many times one has been to the dentist and however gentle she or he might be.

The fear of the needle is another common experience; injections whether as a therapeutic or preventative measure, as at the dentist, when the outcome is beneficial, are not generally liked. Needle phobia in children is very common and can make the administration of analgesics somewhat difficult (P. A. McGrath 1990; Carter 1994). Some people fear the needle at the dentist more than they fear the drill. It is the kind of pain, associated with very sensitive and tender parts, the gums and the inside of the mouth, that seems to make the difference. Shooting or piercing pains can be very unpleasant.

Selye (1956) argued that stress was a response and he described a General Adaptation Syndrome with responses varying from an alarm reaction, to a stage of resistance and then exhaustion. He argued that this is a universal response, unvarying from individual to individual. The only variation is in the strength of the stressor. Lazarus and Folkman (1984) argue however that there is also variation in the appraisal of the stressor by the individual. The meaning of the event for the individual is vitally important to the nature of the response. In the pain situation the importance of the meaning of the situation has a great impact on the individual's reaction to pain. This meaning aspect will be explored in more detail in the next chapter.

Signs and symptoms

Most people will have experienced the signs and symptoms of fear. There may be pallor, particularly of the face, an increased heart beat and pulse rate, increased activity of the sweat glands, creating a cold and clammy feeling. There is usually a dry mouth and difficulty in swallowing, or of talking. The voice may change under the tension and with the dry mouth, becoming more 'squeaky'. There may be increased and shallower breathing, particularly as the tension increases. There are changes to the digestive system, which may lead to feelings of 'butterflies' in the stomach or even nausea and vomiting. There may be a muscular tremor of the hands, or the muscular tension may lead to aches and pains if left untreated for long. The strength of the symptoms will reflect the strength of the stimulus, as perceived by the individual.

Mentally there will be a difficulty in thinking about anything else other than the cause of the anxiety, it will tend to lead to distraction from our day-to-day lives or work situation. There will be difficulty in concentrating, a tendency to make mistakes or to forget things. There may be a withdrawal from other people or from events, or if others do make an effort to help, there will be a tendency to talk about the threatening situation over and over again.

How anxiety works

Cannon (1929) and Baird (1934) proposed what has become known as the Cannon–Baird theory which argues that the information coming into the system stimulates both the physiological and the psychological responses; neither is the precursor of the other. There can in fact be a psychological response without the physiological responses. They also argued that there was the same general physiological response to all emotions. However, that has been criticised by Ekman (1992) and Levenson (1992). They found different responses, although they did find anger and fear to have similar physiological responses. The psychological aspects however seem to vary between individuals depending on the circumstances and their past experiences (Schachter and Singer 1962; Larsen and Diener 1987). In particular the work of Lazarus is important here. These aspects will be discussed more fully in the next chapter.

There is evidence of direct links between the reception of the information and the motor/behavioural responses, bypassing the cognitive processes. This allows an immediate, perhaps survival reaction to occur if the stimulus is very intense or suggests danger (Le Doux 1986). This response seems however to be influenced by the 'mental set' of the individual which relates to the level of trait anxiety (a personality characteristic). State anxiety is the level or kind of anxiety that results from a particular situation or stimulus, as opposed to trait anxiety which is an ongoing level of awareness or sensitivity to anxiety-provoking stimuli.

The stimulus reaching the central nervous system, via the peripheral or special senses, is routed to the thalamus, the hypothalamus and the limbic system, and in particular the amygdala (Le Doux 1986,1989, based on the much earlier work of Papez 1937). In line with the proposals of Cannon–Baird, it seems that the signal goes to the amygdala and to the cortex, in parallel. The amygdala passes the signal on to the sympathetic system if an emotional interpretation is made at that level.

The cortex in the meanwhile provides a more considered interpretation which may confirm or over-ride the initial reading and reaction. Thus we have a kind of emotional reflex action similar to the spinal reflexes, whereby under certain conditions a motor response may be stimulated before there is conscious awareness of the stimulus. However, even then there is the possibility of a cognitive over-ride shortly afterwards. Some neuro-psychological evidence does support the possibility of quick survival responses. The limbic system and the amygdala seem to be important here, helping to assess the emotional significance of a stimulus (Le Doux 1989, 1992; Treede *et al.* 1999).

Arousal, sympathetic and parasympathetic activity

Generally our emotional reactions to events, or even to our own thoughts and imaginings, are related to our level of arousal. This is a phenomenon related to the activity of the sympathetic and parasympathetic nervous systems. The central control of these seems to be placed in the medulla brain stem and the hypothalamus. These are also, as we noted in Chapter 3, involved in the nociceptive processes, being involved in the various stages of the experience of pain, associated with the reticular formation and the limbic system, which, as we now see, are involved with the emotions. The following description of the arousal system, the sympathetic and parasympathetic nervous systems is relatively brief. The reader is referred to specialist textbooks on the nervous system for more detail (e.g. Gale 1986; Green 1987; Hayward 1996).

The ascending reticular activating system (ARAS)

The reticular formation, as well as playing a major part in the experience of pain and in the experience of emotions, is also concerned with the general 'arousal' state of the individual. In this part of the brain is the centre that seems to control the sleep–wake cycle (see, for example, Green 1987; Hayward 1996). Thus all these aspects of experience, being awake, experiencing emotion, pain and also the drive of motivation, are related to activities of this complex area in the central nervous system.

There is a direct relationship between signals from the periphery, messages from the cortical cognitive areas of the brain, and the activating aspects of the ARAS. This activation is achieved by both hormonal and nervous means. The hormonal control is mediated through the secretions of the pituitary gland and in particular the adreno-cortico-trophic hormone (ACTH). The nervous control is mediated through the sympathetic and parasympathetic nervous systems.

The pituitary-adrenal system

The pituitary gland is connected to the hypothalamus by a short stalk, and its activity is related to signals from the hypothalamus, thus achieving co-ordination between nervous and hormonal systems. The pituitary gland, which controls all the endocrine glands including the adrenal cortex, secretes ACTH to stimulate the activity of the adrenal cortex. The adrenal cortex then itself secretes a group of glucocorticoids and mineralocorticoids. Both of these facilitate the preparation of the body for reaction to stress. In particular the glucocorticoids, such as cortisone and corticosterone, are a major component of the body's stress response. They also have a feedback relationship with the anterior lobe of the pituitary gland from which the ACTH is secreted, as well as the hypothalamus and the higher brain centres including the cortex and also the limbic system, where emotional aspects are experienced.

The sympathetic system

The sympathetic system is also associated with the generation of the body's reaction to stimulation, or stress, either from the periphery and external sources or from within, from memories or anticipations of stress. As it is also controlled by the hypothalamus, it acts in correlation with the pituitary-adrenal hormonal system. The sympathetic nervous system controls the adrenal medulla and thus the secretion of adrenaline and noradrenaline. It also controls the activity of the gastro-intestinal system, the circulatory system and the respiratory system. There is some evidence that the sympathetic nervous system, through the activity of noradrenaline, is involved in regenerative changes in the afferent (sensory) nervous system (Baron 1998).

These processes produce a state of alertness and readiness for action. The pupils are dilated, saliva is inhibited (dry mouth), the heart beat is increased, the trachea and bronchi are dilated to improve respiration, digestion is inhibited through the reduction of peristalsis and the secretion of the digestive enzymes. There is increased perspiration which aids cooling of the body in this alert, active state. The blood is stimulated to produce more platelets to facilitate clotting, and there is also increased production of endorphins within the central nervous system.

The parasympathetic system

The parasympathetic nervous system is also controlled by the hypothalamus and is related to the activity of the pituitary-adrenal system. However, it is concerned with maintenance activity within the body. Thus digestion is aided by the production of saliva and the digestive enzymes, and peristalsis is maintained. The heart rate is reduced and the respiratory system also decreases in activity. The tissue-repair processes are stimulated and sugars are converted to fats and stored. The body enters a restful, peaceful stage. Sleep is easier during this phase and after a heavy meal the parasympathetic system is very active. The overall effect then is one of muscular and mental relaxation, while the restorative functions take place.

There are degrees of alertness produced in this way and generally the increase in arousal leads to increased efficiency, particularly with physical activity, but it also affects mental concentration and thinking. However, it seems that as the level of arousal increases there is reached a point where the efficiency decreases and the individual enters a state of panic or can even seem 'paralysed' into inaction. The Yerkes–Dodson law (1908), which describes this inverted 'U' curve of performance, indicates that there must be a certain level of arousal for ordinary activity. As the demand for energy, as in increased speed, effort or accuracy, is increased, then the level of arousal, through the activity of the sympathetic system, is increased. Too much arousal, as in high levels of anxiety and stress, produces loss of control of the energy, and speed, effort and accuracy suffer as a result (Hebb 1955).

Under training and in high performance situations, the improvement in speed effort and accuracy may continue to very high levels, but if pushed too far results in a dramatic loss of speed, effort and accuracy and even a collapse. This has been called the catastrophe theory (Hardy 1988). Selye (1956) has described a General Adaptation Syndrome, consisting of alarm, resistance and exhaustion, and Cannon (1929) very early on identified the arousal mechanism as preparing the body for fright, flight or fight. From the results of an influential experiment, which has however been criticised since, Schachter and Singer (1962) proposed that the particular setting and cognitive response to it by the individual gave rise to a particular emotion. They proposed that this was related to the attributions applied to the situation by the individual. Attributions mean explanations or meanings of the situation according to the person experiencing it and, in particular, causal explanations (see also Chapter 5).

Thus, as the nociceptive signals reach the reticular formation and limbic system an aversive reaction is stimulated. Links with the cortical areas seek information to give meaning to the signals. From this meaning, the particular emotional response is identified, and motivation to do something about the stimulus is generated. Links with the sympathetic and parasympathetic nervous systems lead to the physiological changes that produce the physical symptoms. The more information there is, from other sensory input or from memory, the less uncertainty there will be and the less anxiety and the better coping with the pain situation. The relationship between uncertainty and anxiety was clearly demonstrated recently in a study of women waiting for the results of breast biopsy. However long they had to wait, the women experienced high levels of anxiety, depression, and uncertainty, which were sustained throughout the waiting period (Poole 1998).

The signs and symptoms of anxiety and distress as described above can be helpful in the assessment of pain in situations where there is an inability to indicate the presence of pain verbally, as with the very young infant, or perhaps the very elderly, or those with learning disabilities.

Emotions and pain

Attempts to classify the emotions have been made and one successful one is that of Fischer et al. (1990). They identified two main types, positive and negative. There were sub-categories of these. In the positive group there are love, joy, pride, contentment. In the negative group there are anger, annoyance, hostility and aggression; sadness, grief, depression and guilt; and finally fear and horror. Watson and Clark (1992) identified similar groups in a cross-cultural setting. In this section we shall be considering some of the more common ones associated with pain.

Anxiety and pain

The fears or anxieties may be focused on one aspect of pain, such as surgery. The focus may be on becoming unconscious; waking up during the operation; the actual cutting of the skin (fear of 'the knife'); the outcome of the operation in terms of providing relief from the problem causing the surgery (will it work?); the post-operative pain (how much will it hurt?); scarring from the surgery. There may be fears of mutilation as with surgery to the breast or with the creation of ostomies. The pattern of anxieties will obviously vary from person to person, depending on their previous experience, information gained from friends, relatives, literature including newspapers or films and television (Davis 1984b).

Anxiety, as noted above, is particularly associated with uncertainty of outcome following the anticipation and appraisal of threat or potential threat, for example, prior to surgery or a painful medical intervention (Hayward 1975; Johnson and Vogele 1993). There are also two types of anxiety, state and trait. State anxiety is the reaction to a particular threat or anticipated threat; trait anxiety is a personality trait or a generalised tendency to react in an anxious way. Both types are related to uncertainty.

Anxiety is also a feature of chronic pain. There may be high levels of uncertainty about the future in relation to the course of the disease causing the pain, for example with arthritis (Diamond and Coniam 1991). There may also be uncertainty in relation to the impact of the condition on the individual's lifestyle including employability; the effectiveness of any treatment for the condition or for the pain associated with it (see, for example, Weiner 1985; Roy 1992). The uncertainties may flare up at different times as the various possible sources, ambiguity or lack of information, occur. For example, unexpected changes in the condition, or in the management of the pain, may cause anxiety. Tension and stress are frequent concomitants of chronic pain, and reflect the involvement of the sympathetic nervous system in the pain experience. This can cause pain directly, through muscle tension and headaches, or indirectly by increasing the sensitisation of pain receptors and neurones (see Chapter 3).

There do seem to be some people who develop an increased tendency to 'catastrophise' their situation when experiencing chronic pain. This means that they tend to fear the worst, feeling that they are never going to get better, or that they are going to get worse, and that their lifestyle will deteriorate dramatically (Rosenteil and Keefe 1983; Keefe *et al.* 1989; Vlaeyen *et al.* 1987). This tendency has also been linked with personality characteristics with reference to coping with post-operative pain (Taenzer 1983). There is also evidence that those who do have a tendency to catastrophise are more likely to have higher levels of disability, whatever the level of pain intensity or of depression (Sullivan *et al.* 1998).This separation of catastrophising from depression, as a separate construct, supports the findings of Geisser *et al.* (1994).

The person anticipating surgery, or any acute pain situation, or anticipating the effects of chronic pain or painful interventions, therefore will be experiencing the physiological symptoms of fear and uncertainty, mediated by the sympathetic system. These will include sensations involving the gastro-intestinal tract, dry mouth, butterflies in the stomach, loss of appetite, perhaps a tendency to diarrhoea. There may be cardio-vascular symptoms, or muscular tension and restlessness, and a difficulty in sleeping.

This state is unpleasant in itself and, if severe, warrants some kind of intervention. However, the link between anxiety and the inten-sity of pain has been known for some time. Anticipation of pain increases the reported intensity of pain, and reduction of anxiety decreases the reported intensity of pain (Hill *et al.* 1952; Hall and Stride 1954). Other studies have demonstrated that both state and trait anxiety are related to the intensity of pain reported (e.g. Johnston 1980; Seers 1987). Early nursing research studies as well as more recent ones have demonstrated the benefits of information giving to reduce anxiety and thus the intensity of reported pain, as well as improvement in other post-operative outcomes (Hayward 1975; Boore 1978; Davis 1984a; Johnson and Vogele 1993). The information should include that about sensory aspects, procedural aspects and coping strategies and, if possible, training in these for maximum effect. This will be discussed in more detail in a later chapter.

Anger

Anger can be seen as an emotion that results from a sense of being thwarted in a coping strategy. The individual identifies a way of dealing with the situation but is unable to carry out the process or activity for some reason or factor beyond his or her control. There is a sense of frustration at first which can develop into anger and an aggressive response if the emotional level is increased and there is much energy tied up in the reaction. Some personality types have been proposed as being more likely to exhibit an anger or hostility response to stress than others (Type A). Alternatively they may show defensiveness, negative affect (emotion), and in particular disavowed hostility (Rosenman 1990; Contrada *et al.* 1990), and this has been shown to have deleterious effects on health and ability to cope.

As we have seen in our look at the role of the sympathetic nervous system and emotion, the physical state of arousal with anger is similar to that of fear (Ekman 1992; Levenson 1992). As described above for the action of the sympathetic nervous system, there is the release of energy in preparation of a response and if this cannot be released creatively then it is available for a destructive or at least a negative response. This anger or negative reaction may be turned outwards or inwards, into negative behaviour towards others, or if this is not possible or, as well, self-destructive behaviour towards the individual themselves. If anger cannot be expressed or does not lead to relief from the situation, then repeated experiences of frustration may lead eventually to feelings of helplessness and depression (Beck *et al.* 1985).

Positive emotions

Not all emotions are negative. Some people use humour as an emotional response to stress (Kahn 1989). It provides a mechanism to reframe or review the situation, by trying to see the funny side. Alternatively it is a way of communicating unpleasant or tragic situations or events; self-mocking references to the situation may help the individual to cope. Hostility and anger, which it may not be possible to express, may be converted into humour as an acceptable release. Alternatively a sense of identity may be obtained by making 'in' jokes. It is possible for other positive emotions to be experienced, such as altruism (a concern for and a desire to help others or safeguard them from hurt or anguish), when the situation might seem to demand the expression of anxiety or distress. Alternatively there might be the expression of positive, spiritual emotions such as a love of God and a desire to do His will (Copp 1974) whatever the threat or anticipated suffering associated with the situation. (See the discussion of needs, and in particular Maslow's model (1954), in the section on motivation in this chapter.)

Depression

The person with chronic pain will be particularly prone to depression (Romano and Turner 1985). Chronic pain has such a powerful effect on the whole person, that it can invade all aspects of his or her life and lifestyle. Such people may not be catastrophisers but they will be anticipating or reviewing the long-term implications of the pain, and its relative unmanageability. Their thinking will be dominated by the pain and its implications. This may lead to a sense of low esteem and worthlessness which can have a very marked effect on coping or a desire to participate in rehabilitation.

The experience of depression

Physical and emotional symptoms are common as are cognitive and psychological ones. In this chapter we shall concentrate on the physical-emotional aspects. Physically the patient may feel tired with a loss of appetite, or they might have feelings of restlessness and tearfulness. There my be disruption of sleep with depressed thoughts reverberating in the wakeful periods. A sense of apathy may dominate their approach to life, with perhaps a sense of hopelessness, worthlessness and poor self-esteem. There may be feelings of guilt (Minghella 1992). There seems to be a tendency for women to be more likely to suffer from depression (Haley *et al.* 1985).

There may also be a tendency to cognitive distortions, associated with the depression. There are unrealistic expectations or fears about the situation. The chronic pain sufferer may be concerned about future employment or social relationships; or they may anticipate deterioration in family relationships as he or she anticipates becoming more and more of a burden to the rest of the family (Roy 1992). These thoughts and expectations will reverberate around in the person's mind and reflect back on the depression (Lefebvre 1981). There may be a tendency to attributions of helplessness to the situations as the person reflects on his or her inability to influence events or to cope with the continuing pain or increasing disability. This can lead, some argue, to a state of learned helplessness which is also self-perpetuating (Abramson *et al.* 1978). However, Skevington (1995), in reviewing the literature in this area, suggests that a condition of hopelessness rather than helplessness is a better explanatory model for the link between chronic pain and depression.

The issue of control and controllability in the chronic pain situation seems also to be important.

Depression and pain

Although chronic pain does lead to depression, it does not occur in all people with chronic pain, nor all the time (Romano and Turner 1985). It seems to occur often at times of particular stress, as when there might be a flare-up of the pain, or some implication of the pain becomes more dominant, as there does seem to be a cognitive-behavioural mediation between pain and depression (Turk *et al.* 1995). There does seem to be a tendency for women to report more symptoms of depression than men. This may be because women find it easier to talk about their feelings (Haley *et al.* 1985). Turk *et al.* (1995) also found a tendency for older patients to have depressive symptoms. Skevington (1995) argues that as the symptoms of depression are similar to those of chronic pain, thus it can be difficult to know when there is depression or just a chronic pain syndrome (Black 1975). The assessment process must seek evidence of both.

The depression does seem to be related to the meaning or interpretation of the situation by the sufferer, hence the possible influence of a tendency for distorted or unrealistic interpretations of the situations. Nevertheless, however realistic or unrealistic, the interpretations are always personal and individual, although possibly influenced by family, and social or cultural factors (see Chapter 6). Thus for any particular person suffering from chronic pain there will be an individual reaction, which may include a depressive reaction, and the nature and focus of any depression must be explored with each person being cared for. It does seem that the depression may be related more to the level of disability caused by the pain situation (Peck *et al.* 1989).

There does not seem to be any evidence that a depressive reaction to pain is a personality factor. It seems to be a changeable reaction rather than a fixed personality characteristic. Scores on the depressive scale of personality inventories of people in pain change after treatment (Sternbach 1974), and self-esteem scores improve also after treatment (self-esteem being seen as the opposite of depression; Elton *et al.* 1978). Walding (1991) has suggested an association between depression and a sense of loss or bereavement in the chronic pain situation. This could relate to a sense of a loss of quality of lifestyle.

The physiology of depression

There may be a physiological link between chronic pain and depression. Serotonin is a precursor of the endogenous endorphins and enkephalins. It can also be reduced in depression. Drugs for the treatment of depression such as the tricyclic anti-depressants seem to increase the amount of serotonin which has an analgesic effect as well as an anti-depressant one. The two outcomes have been clearly demonstrated (Monks and Merskey 1984).

Conclusion

Depression is now seen as a natural reaction to a stressor – for example, pain, a realistic and appropriate response, particularly if it becomes long term (Kleinman 1988; Pilowski and Bassett 1982; Melzack and Wall 1996). When measured on tests, such as the Beck Depression Inventory (Beck *et al.* 1988), the scores of people with chronic pain tend to be at the low end of the scale indicating a depressive mood, but not clinical depression. Nevertheless some people in chronic pain do become severely depressed (Doan and Wadden 1989). It is frequently reported in chronic pain, but certainly not always. Reports of depressive symptoms may vary within the same individual as the situation changes (Pilowski and Bassett 1982; Romano and Turner 1985; Skevington 1993).

Thus the person in pain, particularly the person with chronic pain, may report depressive symptoms, dysphoric mood, irritability, loss of energy, fatigue, loss of appetite, concentration, sense of guilt and of being socially undesirable (perhaps because of an inability to play the normal social roles). However, this is not true of every patient. Also the degree of depressive mood will vary from person to person. Nevertheless, it is an important part of the possible pain experience and one that can have serious consequences if not identified.

Motivational aspects of pain

The person experiencing pain is motivated to do something about it, if possible. The obvious example is to avoid or withdraw from the painful stimulus. Another approach is to determine to cope with it if it is impossible to avoid or withdraw. The person then uses a variety of coping strategies. For example, in a study of chronic pain in the elderly, self-determined coping strategies were identified (Walker *et al.* 1990; see Chapter 5).

Even with acute pain in an accident, there is motivation to prevent pain or to prevent further pain. The victim usually is motivated to adopt protective mechanisms such as restriction of movement or weight bearing. The victim will seek help if these protective measures or the self-administration of analgesics do not do the trick or are not feasible. The victim may struggle, limping or crawling for help, in extreme circumstances, enduring much discomfort and even pain in the search for help. This drive can be very powerful. It is related to the arousal that is part of stress and anxiety. It could be seen as the fight part of the stress response, and involves the expenditure of much energy. If unsuccessful and prolonged this drive can absorb so much energy that the person enters into shock, with exhaustion (Selye 1956).

The mechanism of motivation

Motivation can be defined as a complex decision-making process. It enables an animal to move towards a goal (Toates 1986; Epstein 1982).We sometimes talk about goal-directed behaviour. Generally it is associated with feeding, drinking, sex and exploration. It is based on an homeostatic principle to maintain the equilibrium of the internal environment. This is achieved by feedback mechanisms utilising the nervous and hormonal systems, and linked to the activities of the hypothalamus (Roscoe and Myers 1991). The drive is initiated when there is a deficit identified or a need, and this leads to behaviour directed to reducing that deficit (Hull 1952).

For human beings a model that includes more psychological and social goals has been offered by Maslow (1954) who developed a hierarchical model. Rogers (1961) offered a self-actualisation model. Later this approach was developed by Harre (1979), who introduced the social dimension, as did Tajfel (1991). There does seem to be a learning aspect to the psychological and social influences on motivation. In particular this is related to operant conditioning as the individual learns that certain behaviours achieve certain outcomes that may be satisfying their needs (Fordyce 1976). There may even be a social version of the operant conditioning, involving vicarious rewards and role modelling. Effective reinforcers or rewards in this situation have been identified by Turk and Flor (1987). These include direct positive reinforcement such as concern or attention; indirect positive reinforcement, such as escape from responsibilities; negative reinforcement by ceasing certain activities, such as those that increase the pain or make it worse; and negative reinforcement through the non-reinforcement of well behaviours, which tends to increase dependence.

Maslow's model included five levels in hierarchy: physiological, safety, belongingness and love, esteem, and self-actualisation. This model has been criticised as consisting of discrete levels, each of which had to be satisfied before the others could be attempted. However, it is possible to consider overlaps between the levels so that 'higher' levels could be attempted before lower ones were satisfied, or even pre-empting them (Williams and Page 1989; Neher 1991). Thus the individual may deny the satisfaction of physiological needs in order to achieve satisfaction of, say, a safety need or a self-actualisation need. Someone may take a risk to save someone else. Support for the model has been provided by Alderfer (1989) from an organisational study. This does seem to be a useful model for considering the motivational aspects of the pain experience.

Frustration of need or motivation

If the drive to obtain relief from the pain is unsuccessful, frustrated, or prevented from occurring, then a sense of helplessness or hopelessness may develop which will in itself add to the negative feelings associated with the pain experience (Tyrer 1992). Helplessness has been shown to affect motivation to escape and learn from the experience (Abramson *et al.* 1978). This may also be related to a sense of loss and 'bereavement' for a lost lifestyle (Walding 1991). The desire to develop coping mechanisms and to persist in them is related to this motivational aspect of the pain experience.

This sense of being helpless or that the chronic pain situation is uncontrollable by the sufferer has a reciprocal effect on the motivation to cope, or to learn about the situation. It is a perception of the situation by the sufferer and the person will feel like withdrawing from the situation, and become listless and lethargic. There may be feelings of worthlessness and perhaps a sense of loss or bereavement. The symptoms do seem to be similar to those of depression, and the feelings of helplessness may be associated with those of depression. However, the main symptom experienced by the person with the chronic pain is one of not being in control, of being at the mercy of the pain and of others who 'should' or 'ought' to do something about the pain.

Motivation and control

However, the opposite may be experienced by the person with the pain, in that they may feel that they can cope, can do something about the situation, or at least participate. It is a kind of self-confidence. There is a sense of being in control, of being motivated to do something or to comply with recommendations. Some people talk about being challenged by the situation, or being called on by God or other spiritual or personal ethic to cope. There may be comments about a sense of responsibility, or about 'owning the pain'. The person may have had previous experience of the pain. There may be a motivation to find things out, to seek help and support. There may be a willingness to talk to others about the pain and to benefit from others' experiences.

The question of motivation is also related to a sense of self-efficacy (Bandura 1977), and feelings of being in control (Wallston 1989). The person in pain, particularly in chronic pain, may or may not feel in control of things. If the drive to cope with the painful experience is not successful, or is frustrated or means that the sufferer is dependent on others, then the sense of being in control may be lost. However, some people tend to respond to stress by feeling that they can deal with the situation, that they are responsible for their circumstances, that it is up to themselves to do something about things. There are others who tend to feel that they are not responsible, that others, more senior, more qualified, are in control and therefore they must wait until these powerful others 'in control' (and this may include beings such as 'God' or other supernatural entities or forces, even luck) do something about the situation.

Chronic pain by definition is long term. It is understandable that months and years of persisting pain are bound to lead to these symptoms of helplessness, of loss of control, of a sense of excessive dependence on others, of lost quality of life, and a general loss of drive or motivation. This can easily merge with or be a symptom of depression. The motivational and emotional responses to a painful situation are clearly linked, both physiologically and psychologically. Indeed Black (1975) has identified a chronic pain syndrome, which can be self-perpetuating, and which combines depressive symptoms as well as those of helplessness, hopelessness, loss of control and self-efficacy.

Conclusion

In this chapter the experience of pain has been shown to be not only the reception of nociceptive stimuli via the peripheral nervous system, the dorsal horn of the spinal cord, the spinothalamic tracts and the central nervous system. Particularly in the various parts of the central nervous system, such as the limbic system and the reticular formation, are the centres through which physiological and psychological aspects can be experienced which give emotional 'colour' to the pain experience. The combined involvement, in particular, of the meaning given to the stimulus, following cognitive appraisal, together with the activity of the pituitary-adrenal system, the sympathetic nervous system and the parasympathetic nervous system, in relation to that meaning, generates the emotional and motivational reaction to and colouring of the pain experience. In the next chapter we shall explore in more detail the process of giving meaning to the experience through cognitive evaluation of the stimulus.

Chapter 5

Cognitive and evaluative aspects of pain

> the pain that I fancy I feel
>
> Anon

Introduction

In this chapter we discuss those aspects of the experience of pain which are to a certain extent the most visible, or at least, those of which the person experiencing the pain is the most aware. This is the conscious experience of the sensation, whatever it is like for the particular individual, that he or she calls pain. It also includes the expression of the pain. This may be verbal or non-verbal, and the non-verbal may be vocal or behavioural.

Some of the conscious experience has been covered in the previous chapter under the emotional aspects of the experience. To a certain extent, however, the awareness of the emotion and the meaning it gives to the pain experience are dependent on the processes and factors to be considered in this chapter, and helps to create the cognitive-evaluative interpretation of the pain. Also the sensory-discriminatory aspects of the experience are involved in and part of the cognitive-evaluative aspects. Thus it could all seem to be coming together in this chapter. However, we must wait until the next chapter for the full picture, when we look at the social and cultural aspects, which also form part of the cognitive-evaluative.

It can be argued that without conscious awareness, there is no pain. Indeed, this is the argument for the use of anaesthetics in surgery. The patient is rendered unconscious so that there will not be any pain from the actual surgical experience. The pain is experienced however following the return to consciousness when the anaesthetic wears off. Sometimes even sleep can bring some relief from pain, although this usually needs the help of analgesics or sedatives to facilitate the sleep.

To a very large extent we are dependent on the sufferer's conscious experience of pain, his or her cognitive and evaluative assessment of the experience, in order to be able help him or her. According to one definition, it is the person's verbal claim to be in pain that defines the existence of pain (McCaffrey 1968). There is also however, usually (but not always), some evidence of injury or disease or other signs and symptoms to support this claim. There are other definitions related to injury or disease, but as Melzack and Wall have argued, these can be seen as limiting the approach to pain rather than facilitating it (1996; and see Chapter 2).

There are of course particular problems with people who cannot verbalise a claim to be in pain, such as the very young, or the very old, or those with learning difficulties for example. The communication of pain by physiological changes due to the emotional aspects have been considered in the previous chapter, and these changes can be a most helpful resource in identifying and dealing with possible pain in such people. Also some of the non-verbal behavioural aspects of communication to be considered in this chapter are valuable as well.

The patient's experience

As outsiders we usually are aware of someone in pain when they say 'Ouch' or 'That hurts', or there is some other verbal or audible sign (such as a sharply in-drawn breath). As far as the person is concerned, there will be the sense of pain or hurt at the site of the stimulation. This might be the stubbed toe, the operation site, the tooth, the lower back, the lower abdomen, wherever the stimulus for the sensory-discriminative aspect of the experience originated. Depending on the circumstances, there will be some meaning to that experience. In the acute situation this can be fairly straightforward, and the claim to be in pain and the experience of the pain is understandable.

No-one else can know what a particular pain experience is like, even those who have been in a similar situation. In particular the involvement of the motivational-emotional aspects will be very individual, as the person evaluates or appraises the situation and assesses any threat or sense of uncertainty as to the outcome of the situation, particularly with acute pain (Lazarus and Folkman 1984).

With chronic pain the long-term effects of the pain on lifestyle and relationships, as well as what it feels like, will be very dependent on the individual and her or his particular circumstances.

Communication

The intensity, the bearability, the nature of the pain can be communicated to others, especially in words, but also non-verbally and in terms of behaviour. Some of the physiological changes and behavioural responses to the emotional aspects that can occur have been considered in the previous two chapters. Thus signs of anxiety or depression may be shown without there necessarily being words to support them. Such signs can give the carer a clue as to the quality of the experience of the person in pain, and a possible opening for further exploration of that experience. These are the signs described for the activity of the sympathetic nervous system and anxiety (see Chapter 3), together with any signs of injury or disease. From such exploration the meaning and nature of the pain experience can be determined as far as the person can express it. Cognitive-evaluative information about the pain experience is most valuable in helping the carer to be able to provide the most apt and efficacious help.

To start with, descriptions of the position or site of the pain, any movement of the pain, or its extent can be given. These will vary from individual to individual and with the nature of the pain experience (Melzack and Torgerson 1971). The kind of pain can be described also, such as any burning, shooting or piercing aspects to it. It might be described as an ache rather than a pain. It may be deep or superficial, it may be personalised and given human characteristics, particularly negative ones, such as being vicious, evil or sneaky. It will also be given some emotional or motivational attributes, such as worrying, frightening or depressing, or be described as making the person want to give up, or declare that he or she is not going to be beaten. The effect of the pain on the sufferer's lifestyle may be expressed, with reference to work, to relationships, to their own expectations of themselves (Roy 1992).

Acute pain

There will be different kinds of words and meanings expressed in the acute and chronic pain situations. With acute pain, the emphasis will be on verbalising the sensation and intensity, indicating the site and range of the pain. There may be tears or cries of pain. Expressions of anxiety about the seriousness of the situation may be made, or about the likely outcome. There may be appeals for relief. In the post-operative situation, if the pain is worse than expected there may be some expressions of resentment, or even anger. However, there may also be an acceptance of the pain as a sign that the pain or suffering of the original disease or problem would be removed as a result of the surgery. The patient may claim to be able to cope, or even be willing to cope with pain as part of the treatment (removal of stitches or drains), or the rehabilitation process as he or she undergoes physiotherapy for example. It will be possible for the carer to enter into a discussion with the sufferer as to strategies for care or rehabilitation.

If the pain results from an accident there may be expressions of responsibility, or guilt, 'if only I hadn't ... '. Alternatively there may be expressions of anger if the sufferer feels that he or she is the victim of someone else's mistake. If the treatment of the injury is going to take a long time, and consequently the possibility of pain continuing (such as with extensive lacerations, burns, or complicated fractures), then there may be a depressive reaction, compounded with anxiety about the outcome. The possibility of scarring or loss of function will complicate the reaction and influence the response to the pain. Again the meaning of the pain for the person is important in planning a care or rehabilitation programme.

Chronic pain

With chronic pain there are obvious links, also, with the motivational-emotional aspects as the person in pain gives utterance to the feelings being experienced, which are related to their appraisal of the situation (Lazarus and Folkman 1984). However, as indicated above there will be much individual variation in the reaction and in the way in which this is verbalised. The longer the pain continues without much relief or promise of relief, then the more the sufferer will be concerned with coping in the long term, with the impact on his or her quality of life. These may be couched in terms of depression, as a negative view is taken of the future and the possibility of permanent relief. This may be expressed as helplessness or hopelessness, and be linked with a failure to cope (Seligman 1975; Beck 1976). The latter may

involve a reluctance to continue with or even start or initiate reha-
bilitative procedures.

Arguments may be made about the hopelessness of the situation.
The professionals may be accused of not trying, with anger and
frustration coming to the fore. The anger or frustration may be
directed at the cause of the injury or disease that has caused the
pain, such as an employer, the person who caused an accident or
even God as the cause of the situation. There may be a handing
over to the professionals, a rejection of personal responsibility for
the future (Affleck *et al.* 1987). The perceived grim future may then
be blamed on the professionals. Such a passive role-taking may be
reflected in changes to the lifestyle and relationships of the patient.
This may lead to a very restricted life, with increased dependence on
others.

The depressive reaction may be more self-punitive, with a sense
of personal responsibility for the pain, with self-blame or regrets being
uttered. This may lead to attempts to change behaviour in order to
correct the situation. Alternatively there may be a deeper depression
and a sense of worthlessness and of being a failure, 'if only I hadn't
....' or 'why didn't I ... ', or 'if only I had listened to ... '.

Motivation

Some people react to situations like this by having a positive sense
of responsibility to do something about it. There may be expressions of needing to cope, of being in control and of involvement
with the professionals in determining what is done about the pain.
There may be positive changes to the lifestyle in order to facilitate
rehabilitation. The person with such an approach to his or her
chronic pain may initiate their own coping strategies (Walker *et al.*
1990). Even if not generating his or her own response in this way
there may be more of a willingness to participate in a professionally
developed programme of rehabilitation, or set of coping strategies.

Some patients with a positive approach may see the pain as being
character building or as a chance to prove themselves, perhaps in
some religious way. This can be seen sometimes in patients from, for
example, Islamic cultures, where the challenge of the pain is seen as
bringing the patient closer to God. This sense of fighting the pain,
or seeing the pain as something to be overcome, can be expressed by
patients with a terminal condition, such as cancer. This is another
situation where the patient may be able to initiate or follow coping

strategies, drawing on their religion or other spiritual resources. There might also be a cultural dimension to this (see Illich 1976; Helman 1994; Davis 1998). Also however there can be the opposite as the pain is compounded by the thoughts of death. Here the ability to see themselves as being able to cope may be too much and a sense of helplessness and futility, of hopelessness and of being deserted, may overpower the sufferer (Abramson *et al.* 1989). In such situations there may be very little expressed by the patient, who may remain apparently withdrawn and quiet, listless, not responding to enquiries.

In some cases there may be an outspoken desire to end it all, or for the end to come soon. There might be a great deal of distress and emotional expression at the unfairness of it all. This might mean weeping and crying. The anguish may lead to verbal expressions of anger, frustration or swearing as the strain of the continual pain, together with the impending death, becomes too much for the sufferer. This may perhaps be projected onto the staff, or against God or some other entity, even onto the person him or herself, or the pain itself, as a separate being almost. The pain may be seen as wicked or evil in the way it resists treatment; as a bully or a being that is attacking them. The patient may feel that they are being punished or tortured as he or she seems to get little or no respite from the pain.

The words used to describe the situation may become almost poetic as the patient attempts to put into words these kinds of feelings about the pain and about the meaning of the situation for him or her (Melzack and Torgerson 1971).

Special aspects

There may be times when the person in pain gives a picture verbally that is at odds with his or her physical or physiological signs. They may underplay the pain, claiming that it is not too bad, or even non-existent, and yet there may be obvious physical signs of damage, injury or disease, for example as described in the seminal paper by Beecher (1959). This may occur at times of great stress or motivation to overcome the pain, for a variety of reasons, such as helping someone else, or to satisfy some religious or cultural imperative. Women may belittle the pain of childbirth because of their desire to give birth, and yet at the same time acknowledge that it is a painful procedure. In relatively rare circumstances some individuals cannot feel pain, through conditions causing sensory paralysis, or even more rarely through being born without the ability to feel pain (Sternbach 1968)

In other situations someone may complain of being in pain and yet it may be difficult for the professionals to identify any cause for the pain. Some headaches are of this nature, and phantom pain, usually associated with amputation, is another example (Schoenen *et al.* 1994; Jensen *et al.* 1985). In other situations the patient may continue to complain of pain when to all intents and purposes the professionals feel that the original injury or disease has been healed or cured. This is particularly common with lower back pain, when there may be no clinical signs of damage or disease to warrant the complaint, or signs of deterioration in the condition. Some diseases of the nervous system can cause intense or long-lasting pain, and yet the clinical signs of disease or damage may be difficult to identify, for example with trigeminal neuralgia or post-herpetic shingles (e.g. Scadding 1994). Yet in all of these situations the experience of the pain is most real and intense to the sufferer. It can be described clearly and graphically, including its position and movement, its nature and bearability. It may be associated also with behavioural changes or restrictions in movement.

The process of giving meaning to experiences

How do the kinds of meanings of, or reactions to, pain that have been mentioned above occur? If we can understand the psychological processes that lie behind them, it should be easier for us to be able to interact more effectively and to devise more effective interventions. As well as feelings about pain in terms of emotional reactions or responses, we have thoughts about the pain, which can interact with the emotions of course. It is these thoughts and meanings, linked with the emotions, that give rise to behaviour.

It would seem that from birth we are busily interpreting the information that we receive via our sense organs, including proprioception and internal sensations. The information is focused through the attention that we pay to it. There are various models of this process. One is called the information-processing model (Case 1985). Another is the Piagetian model based on the work of Piaget who looked at the ways that the developing infant, child, adolescent, adult create representations about the world he or she lives in (1983). The final model is that based on the work of Vygotsky who argued that the information received by the individual is essentially gained from other people, that cognitive development and activity is essentially a social phenomenon (1962). These models will be presented in more detail in the section on cognitive development in children below. Meadows (1993) has extensively reviewed these. We only have space for a brief review of the essentials of each of these. However, it is hoped that by such a comparison of the main models we can obtain a picture of the cognitive-evaluative processes involved in the pain experience.

The main point of all the models is that information is received by the individual, through the senses including the special senses. There is a selection process by means of which we pay attention to only certain of the kinds of information coming in. We seem to have in-built systems to handle the information, by means of which we can recognise the material, store it and link different sets of information with each other and build up complicated 'pictures' or representations of our experience in a variety of sensory modalities. From these and through other processes we can develop and use strategies for action in response to the information received, or proactively when we initiate behaviour.

What the processes create or deal with

Our cognitive activity deals with units of information which are linked together because of certain aspects that they have in common. They are clustered together into various categories and hierarchies of categories. These create abstract representations of the world and our relationship with it, and links between these facilitate action and behaviour or ways of dealing with the information.

Concepts

The linked and categorised units of information are known as concepts. These categories are based on common features perhaps related to sets of ideal features (Rosch et al. 1976; Bourne et al. 1979). The concepts are related to the level of cognitive activity that is operating. Thus a sensori-motor concept will be different from an emotional one, and from a cognitive one. However, these different concepts may be linked to produce higher-order representations and this may comprise both concrete and abstract qualities (Collins and Quillan 1970).

Thus we have the concrete sensori-discriminative and the abstract cognitive-evaluative meaning, linked by a mixture of concrete physiological and abstract meaning of the emotional aspect of the pain. Rosch *et al.* (1976) have proposed the idea of a hierarchy of concepts.

Schemata

Piaget (1978) used the word schema to describe a representation which is developed and modified as a result of experience through assimilation and accommodation. The experience may involve information from other people. Thus a schema for 'car' will involve a variety of concepts: concrete concepts (a physical car and its physical parts) together with abstract concepts about mobility, speed, safety, travelling from A to B. Generally schemata are about using information, categorised into hierarchies of concepts, in order to achieve a goal.

Schemata were described by Bartlett as long ago as 1932 as comprising past experiences (memories) and their associated meanings. Rumelhart (1980) proposed schemata as plays, theories, computational procedures or analytical procedures, and Baron and Byrne (1984) emphasised social schemata relating to roles, the self and personhood. Another term used in a similar context is script, which is much more related to playing out an action or a social situation (Schank and Abelson 1977).

Constructs

Other words used in the context are construct and construing (Kelly 1955, 1991). Construing is the process of creating interpretations or definitions of aspects of the world and our life in it. The interpretation, or defining characteristic of the entity or element being construed, is known as a construct. Constructs therefore create a personal theory, or expectation as to what is 'out there'; they form 'the inside story', a personal view. This then allows us to plan ahead, have expectations about people, situations or things, and to act accordingly (Fransella 1995). This model or process is dealt with in much more detail in Chapter 6, where it is considered in the context of social relationships.

Similarly, Johnson-Laird (1983) proposed that we create mental models of aspects of the world and our life in it, based on experience and previous knowledge. The personal meaning of the model is what is important, often socially determined through our relationships with others, individuals or groups (Braine *et al.* 1984). One of the most important concepts is that of self, what we think we are like ourselves. This relates to the esteem with which we hold ourselves and the potential which we see for ourselves (Rogers 1961). It also involves a sense of ability to cope with various aspects of our life, our self-efficacy (Bandura 1977). This affects our thought processes, problem solving, persistence in pursuing goals, decision making when choices have to be made, and dealing with uncertainty and stress.

Conclusion

In summary then it seems that the consensus view of what we deal with when we think about things or situations is information about the world and our place in it, gained through our senses and including information from other people. This information is clustered or categorised into meaningful units which enable us to use the information to interact with the world. The units are related to each other as hierarchies, and include sensori-motor information, and information about ourselves such as our emotions. They can be imaginary, dealing with our plans for the future, our hopes and fears, as anticipatory schemata.

Generally these meaningful units are action or goal orientated and the meaning relates to the value or importance of the schema in the achievement of the goal. The hierarchies of concepts relate to the hierarchy of needs as expressed by Maslow (1954; see Chapter 4). If the schema relates to the non-achievement of a goal then it will have a negative meaning. The meaning, positive or negative, usually reflects emotional aspects of the schema, as well as other aspects. It will also reflect social aspects of the situation. Because much of the information we receive, particularly at the higher-order levels, is verbal from our family, friends, colleagues or other sources, language is an important medium for thinking about things, and for our own communications with others about what is happening or important to us.

The role of learning

We have been discussing the development of representations of the world and our life in it, and of strategies and procedures for dealing with it. This has involved taking in new information and modifying old knowledge and ways of dealing with situations. Learning can be defined as a more-or-less permanent change in behaviour or behavioural potential, as a result of experience (Westen 1996). We have therefore been implying the role of learning, if not explicitly mentioning it.

Briefly, there are seen to be three kinds of learning: that resulting from operant or (more rarely) classical conditioning; that resulting from cognitive activity; and that resulting from observation, or modelling, which can be seen as a type of cognitive or social learning.

Conditioning

Conditioning accepts the principle that changes in behaviour come about as a result of the reinforcement of the new behaviour. With classical conditioning, innate responses become associated with a neutral stimulus which has been paired with an unconditioned stimulus (which provokes the innate response without any learning being required). This is important with regard to emotional responses (see the classical work of Pavlov (1927), and Watson and Rayner (1920); and for an up-to-date overview Hayes (1994)). Operant conditioning depends on some kind of reward (which can be described as satisfaction of a need or drive) or punishment to change the behaviour (see the classical work of Thorndyke (1931), and Skinner (1971); and, for example, Westen (1996)). The behaviour has to occur first however, hence the name 'operant'.

Reward can be positive or negative. Positive reward occurs when something desired is gained; negative reward occurs when something not wanted is removed through the continuation of the behaviour. Punishment occurs with the application of something not wanted or the removal of something in order to bring about the cessation of some kind of behaviour. Both kinds of reinforcement have been shown to be effective with regards to behaviour, although there have been problems with punishment as a means of changing behaviour (MacIntyre and Cantrell 1995). It has been shown to lead to further, but different, undesirable behaviour such as withdrawal, aggression or deceit. It also has been shown to lead to only temporary changes in behaviour, until the punishment or threat of punishment is removed.

If an individual fails to find a way of behaving that will bring about the removal of some unwanted stimulus, then a situation known as learned helplessness may occur. Seligman (1975) related this tendency to the apathy of depression and Abramson *et al.* (1978) suggested that the learned helplessness resulted from the way in which those involved gave meaning to the situation. They proposed that this results from a depressive attributional style. This implies that there must be this depressive tendency prior to any learned helplessness occurring. The evidence for this would seem to be inconclusive, particularly in relation to pain (Skevington 1995).

Cognitive learning

Cognitive learning is related to the discussion above, of information processing, concept and schemata formation and development, and problem solving (see the early work of Kohler (1925) and what he called 'insight learning' and Tolman (1932 and 1948) with his 'cognitive maps'; and Hayes (1994) for a more up-to-date overview). The learning that occurs in this situation may not be directly related to environmental stimuli. The solution to a problem may be dealt with in the 'abstract' first prior to being tried out. The individual reformulates representations of the situation (the schemata), and can try out new approaches. This process may not be conscious and the solution may seem to occur out of the blue. The process can often be facilitated by others, in what is known as observational or social learning.

Observational or social learning

Observational or social learning results from watching the behaviour of others in the same or similar situations, who act as models (Bandura 1971, 1977). According to Bandura four processes are involved. Attention must be paid to the model; there must be internalisation of the behaviours, in terms of memory and formulation or reformulation of our own schemata; there must be the ability and/or skill to carry out the new behaviour; and finally there must be a desire to repeat the modelled behaviour. This depends on the perception of reward or success accruing from the behaviour by the model, or the esteem or respect we hold for the person showing the behaviour. This is a form of imitation, which can also be seen as a form of social learning.

People involved in helping others learn new skills or ways of coping often incorporate both operant conditioning and modelling techniques to help the neophyte to move more quickly through the skill levels (Wood *et al.* 1976). This is known as scaffolding.

Attributions

The way in which we try to explain to ourselves what is happening to us and around us is called making attributions (Heider 1958). In particular they relate to the causes of situations, and we tend to prefer stable (repeatable) causes rather than unstable (unpredictable) causes. The theory of attributions is mainly relevant to social relationships, and our perceptions of people doing things to us. Intentionality is a major characteristic (Jones and Davis 1965). Also attributions may be dispositional (something in the individual made them behave that way), or situational (circumstances beyond the person's control made them behave that way).

One issue relating to attribution theory is that of the fundamental attribution error. By this is meant the tendency to attribute dispositional causes to others and yet situational causes to ourselves (e.g. Nisbett *et al.* 1973; Ross *et al.* 1977; Gilbert and Mulkay 1984). Although there is strong evidence in support, this can lead to blaming others ('it's not my fault, he, she or they should have ... ') (Frazier 1990), or a self-serving bias ('I couldn't help it, I was suffering from ... ') (Brown and Rogers 1991). If attempting to see things from the other's perspective, however, then the attributions change or are less dispositional (Storms 1973).

In determining whether or not a dispositional attribution is to be made or not, we tend to take three aspects of the situation into account (Kelley 1967, 1973). These are consistency, consensus and distinctiveness. Consistency is concerned with how regularly the behaviour occurs; consensus refers to whether or not others behave in the same way; and distinctiveness is concerned with the focus of the behaviour, does it only occur with such and such a person or situation? However, Lalljee (1981) argued that other factors have to be taken into account as well. Is the person aware of the behaviour that is expected? What is the relationship between the participants in the situation? The focus or topic of the situation is also important. Finally what are the likely social consequences of the situation? Both of these authorities, however, neglect to emphasise the importance of the individual's way of seeing the world and others in it. Their motives and constructs, their schemata, will be very individual and the general processes identified by Kelley and Lalljee (see above) for example will be interpreted and modified in the light of those personal aspects (Kruglanski *et al.* 1983).

Lazarus (1991), in his cognitive motivational-relational theory of emotion, argues that the attributions made in the appraisal of a potential threat play an important part of our emotional response (see also Chapter 4). The motivational aspect refers to the current drive to do something about the situation. The cognitive appraisal of the situation assesses its meaning to the individual. He described primary and secondary appraisal. The first refers to the assessment of the relevance of the situation to personal goals, its potential effect on self-esteem and personal commitments. Secondary appraisal relates to responsibility, blame or credit, coping potential, whether the future of the situation will lead to improvement or deterioration. The emotional outcomes from such an appraisal, for example, could be anxiety if there is uncertainty; shame if a sense of personal failure is the result of the appraisal; sadness if loss is identified.

Lazarus and Folkman (1984) claim that there is a transactional process between the individual and these aspects. Thus the relationship between the individual and the environment, its meaning to the individual, is vital. The concepts and schemata generated or reformulated as a result of the constant appraisal and re-appraisal then are embodied in the responses to the situation. Thus emotions are seen as processes rather than fixed responses, which are related to the drives, motives and goals of the individual. They result from cognitive activity and relate to the physiological responses stimulated by the situation, as mentioned in the previous chapter. Uncertainty can be appraised as threat or opportunity. The physiological response of the sympathetic nervous system can energise either reaction, depending on the cognitive evaluation.

Moscovici (1984) identified social attributions or representations that reflect societal beliefs and explanations and these will be considered further in the next chapter, when we look at social and cultural aspects of pain.

Cognitive evaluation and pain

With regard to representations of illness and the self as being ill, Leventhal *et al.* (1984) have explored the kinds of schemata developed and the processes involved. They describe an information-processing system, involving active, parallel processing of information. They argue that there are stages in the processing and that it is hierarchical (Leventhal 1982; Leventhal and Mosbach 1983). From these processes the attributes of illness representations are created: identity of the illness; its cause; the consequences; and the duration.

Patients monitor their bodily symptoms and come to a diagnosis; alternatively, given a label they will tend to find the symptoms (Leventhal *et al.* 1980; Meyer 1981). This can lead to treatment-seeking behaviour, but may also lead to self-determined regimes for treatment. However, this will vary from illness to illness, for example it is different for blood-pressure problems and cancer (Meyer 1981), and Pennebaker *et al.* (1981) suggest that the choice of internal or external cues can influence the accuracy of self-diagnosis.

Ciccone and Grzesiak (1984) have identified eight types of schemata created or used by people with chronic pain. There is the awful nature of the experience; being under external control; mislabelling somatic sensations; cognitive rehearsal; the importance of self-efficacy; immediate gains rather than those in the longer term; poor opinion of self; injustice. The creation or formulation of schemata depends very much on the situation as interpreted by the individual. Expectations are important (Anderson and Pennebaker 1980) in labelling the symptoms or feelings. Pain schemata can be more clear or memorable than others (Morley 1993), consisting of all sensory information including social factors and personal meaning (Katz and Melzack 1990). They are particularly vulnerable to the media, as are many illness representations. These may not be medical diagnoses, but they influence the behaviour (Leventhal *et al.* 1988).

The role of learning, particularly conditioning, has been proposed by Fordyce (1976, 1984). This relates especially to the role of gains from pain behaviour (Bokan *et al.* 1981). A learned pain syndrome has been identified by Brena and Chapman (1985). This includes dramatisation; disuse; drug misuse; dependency; disability, and echoes the model proposed by Karoly and Jensen (1987). The role of modelling in influencing pain behaviour has been demonstrated by, for example, Fagerhaugh (1974) and Craig (1978). Strong support for this approach is gained from the efficacy of therapeutic interventions based on the same principles (Keefe 1982; Turner and Romano 1984; Peters and Large 1990).

Cognitive theories of learning have also been influential in the study of pain. Here there is an overlap with the work on the development of schemata and representations of the pain situation. The learning theorists argue for the possibility of change through cognitive activity. Thus information has led to the creation of the schemata or representations, and so further information or new ways of construing the situation can be effective in creating new, more positive, therapeutic schemata (see Chapter 6).

The interrelatedness of emotions, motivation and cognition are seen as vital to the process. Thus anxiety (Bolles and Franslow 1980); depression (Beck *et al.* 1979); coping style (Cohen 1987); self-efficacy (Bandura 1977); locus of control (Rotter 1966); memory (Pincus *et al.* 1993); and personal construing (Kelly 1955, 1991), although studied individually in relation to pain, could all be inter-related with each other into a complex multi-factorial model. Certainly in assessing the pain experience in any individual all of these factors are of value.

The meaning of pain

Thus we have the creation of an individual, personal set of meanings for the sufferer. Fordham and Dunn (1994) have proposed three main types of meaning. The first are philosophical and religious meanings. The big questions such as why me? why now? are asked and meaning sought through attempts to find answers to them. This can also be a way of coping with intractable and severe pain. There may be social and cultural influences here, as argued by Illich (1976), Helman (1994) and Davis (1998), whereby internalised answers from religious sources may be of great value. This is supported by findings from interviews by Copp (1974).

The second kind of meanings are biological. Here the meaning of warning is embodied in a current international definition of pain (IASP 1979). However, as we have noted above, some pains do not seem to be related to any symptom or sign of disease or injury. Alternatively, the pain may be much too late in the progress of a disease to be a warning. This is particularly the case in chronic pain. It is difficult to see the value of such pain, other than perhaps in terms of the philosophical or religious meanings. The third kind of meanings are the social meanings or consequences of pain. These will of course be very individual. We shall be considering social and cultural aspects of pain in the next chapter.

However, there can be seen to be a fourth kind of meaning of pain, and that is the meaning given to the individual as self-knowledge gained through the way in which they cope with the experience. The self-concept is one of the main concepts created in the process of cognitive development. It plays a major role in the outcome of the pain experience. We have considered some aspects of it above in looking at self-esteem, attributions of responsibility and self-efficacy for example. An awareness of the changing, developing nature of the self-concept must play an important part in planning care

Self-efficacy and control

The appraisal of the self and the situation is related to control and coping. Self-efficacy is an important part of motivation too (Bandura 1977). The sense of control is seen as being two dimensional, either an external locus or an internal locus (Rotter 1966). Some argue that a positive appraisal of self is more important than sense of control (Wallston 1989; Victor *et al.* 1986).

Bandura (1977) proposed certain requirements or influences on self-efficacy: previous experience or performance; observation of the experience in others; verbal persuasion through others; and a good physiological status, feeling fit and strong. Self-efficacy is seen as being a changeable state, not a personality factor (Lorig *et al.* 1989). Bandura (1991) claims that a greater level of self-efficacy will lead to a greater persistence in handling stressors; a greater tendency to seek information and/or skills; more positive feelings; and a tendency to view unpleasant aspects more positively. It is argued that a lack of self-efficacy can lead to feelings of helplessness, withdrawal, lethargy and perhaps guilt and anxiety, and that this can be a major component of depression (Seligman 1975; Beck 1976).It is also related to the evaluation of the situation as being one of loss of control. Skevington (1993) argues however that the sense of helplessness and self-blame follow depression.

There is evidence of a relationship between locus of control and pain. An increased belief in chance or external control has been associated with a greater intensity of pain and frequency of pain (Toomey *et al.* 1991). Alternatively, a greater sense of internal control has been associated with a lower intensity and frequency of pain (Bowers 1968; Kanfer and Seidner 1973). Those with a sense of internal control, who have no opportunity to exercise it however, may have to revert to external control with effects on their reaction to the pain situation (Affleck *et al.* 1987). People may also volunteer or hand over control to others when it is felt that the 'expert' knows best (Deci and Ryan 1987).

Cognitive development and the meaning of pain in children

Understanding how children perceive and give meaning to illness in general and to pain in particular is an important aspect of the assessment and care of their pain experience. Gaining access to the adult's pain experience is difficult enough even when we share the same language. When it comes to children, this becomes a major dilemma. They may not have the same vocabulary, use it in the same way, or be as articulate in describing their pain sensations.

The Piagetian model has been mentioned briefly above, and in spite of many criticisms, still holds sway, as does the importance of communication and relationships as argued by Vygotsky, and the processing of information. Following a more detailed presentation of these models, there will be a brief consideration of children's understanding of health, illness and pain, and the presentation of an approach to the utilisation of this information (Davis and Dreliozi 1996).

Information processing

The information-processing model is related to computer functioning and generally assumes a linear process (see, for example, Case 1985; Kail and Bisanz 1982). This model seems to work well when straightforward rules can be operated linking input to output, as say in playing chess. The main aspects to this model are the storage, retrieval and handling of information. The handling of the material is thought to involve goal setting, searching, evaluating, retagging or relabelling, and consolidation of the outcomes.

More recent models however take guidance from insights into the way in which the brain is structured and seems to function; in other words they have a biological approach rather than a mechanistic, computer approach (McClelland *et al.* 1986). These models argue that there might be parallel processing, networks of links or connections between different aspects of the information-processing system. This would seem to echo what we know of the way the individual works and examples of neuronal functioning we have considered in the previous chapters. There are no 'stores' of information, knowledge or memories as such in particular locations, but links between different sets of information which when stimulated reveal the particular knowledge or memory or meaning (McClelland *et al.* 1986; Clark 1989).

The Piagetian model

This is now very well established but much criticised and modified, and has influenced much educational and child-rearing behaviour as well as giving insight into adult cognitive behaviour (Donaldson 1978; Piaget 1983). Piaget proposed a series of developmental stages or phases for cognitive development, tied to specific ages. These are sensori-motor, which is perhaps self-explanatory; pre-operational; concrete operational, which relates to concrete things or events; and formal operational, which relates to abstract thoughts about things or events, or even thoughts about thoughts. What is meant by thoughts is discussed below.

More recent formulations of the model see the process as being much less of steps occurring at particular ages but as a steady flow of development with the various levels of development merging one into another or over-lapping each other. It does not seem either that the earlier levels are lost or over-written, but are subsumed as part of the later or higher levels of cognitive activity (Donaldson 1978; Case 1992).

The Piagetian (1983) model is very much an abstract model describing information processing which could apply in any structure or with any content. The major contribution, other than that of the phases of development, is that of the processes by which information is handled. This involves assimilation, accommodation and equilibration. Assimilation is the process by which new information is related to pre-existing knowledge or understanding. Thus new information can be recognised, and interpreted or modified in the light of what is already known or understood, and creates schemata (see below). Accommodation is the process whereby new information causes changes in the existing knowledge or understanding. Equilibration refers to the necessity of maintaining a sense of coherence or consistency in the developing knowledge and understanding. Thus new information coming in which contradicts the existing views of the world or ideas will lead to an internal adjustment to regain equilibrium, or to changes in behaviour which will change the information coming in.

Piaget also considered the role of action or interaction with the environment as important, especially the social environment. Language and symbolic representation are also important as is the ability to see things from someone else's point of view, decentring.

To a certain extent the individual can cope with a certain amount of inconsistency or contradiction between sets of knowledge or between understandings, perhaps by developing a higher order of understanding which can absorb and accept the contradictions. For example, we can still love someone who has aspects of their behaviour that we dislike, or we can continue to go to work in spite of sometimes very negative aspects to it. We can learn to live with a certain degree of pain by developing a different view of the pain and other aspects of our life. If it is difficult or impossible to achieve equilibrium with respect to some aspect of our life then this will lead to anxiety and stress. Equilibrium can be seen perhaps as achieving a solution to contradictions or inconsistencies (Piaget 1978).

Vygotsky's model

Some solutions, whilst achieving equilibrium, may not be as successful as others in a given situation. Vygotsky's model (1962) emphasises the influence of other people on the development of knowledge, understanding and strategies for dealing with the world. It shows a way in which the individual can not only develop knowledge and understanding but also be shown better solutions by others. Parents, friends, teachers and other significant others can thus 'educate' the individual to more or less successful ways of assimilating, accommodating and achieving equilibrium.

Vygotsky (1986) and his followers propose that this is the main way in which cognitive development occurs. They argue that communication with other people is the main way in which information is received and from which the concepts and schemata can be built. Nevertheless the individual is also receiving information directly from their own interactions with other aspects of the environment. This model certainly makes a better case for the development of more advanced levels of cognitive activity from less advanced ones. An important part of this process of social influence is language whereby meanings as well as knowledge or strategies can be transmitted from one to another. It is through the incorporation of language into our mental processes that we can achieve an adaptive control of thought (ACT, or Adaptive Control Theory, Anderson 1983). This occurs through interlinked propositions, or combinations of mental and verbal images (Paivio 1991). Figure 5.1 shows the main points of each of these models for comparison.

Children's perception of health and illness

There is some evidence that children's perceptions of their health and/or illness develop in a way that reflects cognitive development (Bibace and Walsh 1980; Brewster 1982). Much of the research has been based on models of the generation and growth of causal relations. Children have been interviewed using a series of questions constant across subjects. Probes were used if the responses were vague, sparse or unclear. The following kinds of explanations were found: pre-logical, utilising phenomenism (the allocation of a cause to a distant

Piagetian	Information processing	Social interaction and language
Assimilation of information to existing schemata	**Storage** of multi-modality information	**Internalisation** of experiences in social situations

Accommodation of existing schemata to new information	**Retrieval** and **handling** by parallel processing involving:
	 • goal setting
	 • searching
	 • evaluating
	 • re-labelling
	 • consolidation within a framework of:
	   • self-monitoring
	   • automatisation
	   • detection of consistencies and inconsistencies
		Symbolic representations of reality including **language** which facilitates social interaction by **'scaffolding'** and providing social developmental support for individual development

Decentring: moving from a more egocentric to other centred view		
All helping to achieve a state of		
Equilibrium or balance with the environment		

Figure 5.1   A comparison of models of cognitive development

phenomenon) and contagion (the allocation of a cause to some-thing or someone nearby, physically close); concrete-logical, utilising contamination (by physical contact or the performance of a contami-nating act), and internalisation (the cause is taken inside the body, by inhaling or swallowing); formal-logical involving abstract concepts about the structure and functioning of the body and illness-inducing factors.

Children's perception of pain

Much research has failed to demonstrate clear developmental patterns in pain perception by children. Nevertheless children have been shown to be able to communicate their pain experience well. Hospitalisation or previous pain experience have been shown to influ-ence the perception of pain. Children see pain as a bad thing and seem to be unaware of any good aspects to pain, for example as a warning signal (e.g. Eland and Anderson 1977; Savendra *et al.* 1982).

However, one study in particular has shown developmental patterns in the perception of pain by children (Gaffney and Dunne 1986). They describe the following stages: concrete definitions, describing pain as a thing or a place that hurts or as the result of some action; semi-abstract definitions, describing pain as a feeling or a sensation, but in relation to an unpleasant physical quality, or by the use of synonyms; and finally abstract definitions, usually involving the use of physiological or psychological terms. There is a tendency to use a larger range of themes in describing the pain, which reflect an increasing understanding of the biological purpose of pain, and its relationship to illness and trauma, as well as to the psychological and sociological aspects (Abu-Saad 1984).

Although these stages could be clearly identified as types of response, it was also found that individual children might give responses belonging to two adjacent stages. In this way the more cognitively developed child might give responses reflecting his or her advanced cognitive level, but also responses from earlier levels as well. Gaffney and Dunne (1986) argue that the reasons for their strong developmental patterns include: a sample ranging in age over those ages generally seen as covering the Piagetian stages, and also school stages; a higher age limit of 14 years; and a more sensitive data-collection method allowing a variety of themes to be identified from the children's responses (see Figure 5.2 for a summary of the types of perceptions of health and illness and of pain).

Illness	Pain
Pre-logical • phenomenism • contagion (human action)	*Concrete* • a thing or a place hurts or the result of an action hurts
Concrete-logical • contamination • internalisation (physical action)	*Semi-abstract* • a feeling or sensation in relation to an unpleasant physical experience • the use of synonyms
Formal-logical • abstract concepts (multiple causes and interactions)	*Abstract* • the use of physiological or psychological explanations

Figure 5.2   Children's explanations of illness and pain

In the light of the evidence and models presented above, there are obvious implications for the assessment and management of pain in children. It is vitally important that consideration is given to the level of an individual child's cognitive development and to those factors that can influence the way in which the child might deal with the pain situation. This is considered in more detail in Chapter 10.

Conclusion

In this chapter we have considered the ways in which information is received by the individual, particularly that from internal sources, but also that from the external world. This information is stored as structured hierarchies of clustered information which enables the individual to give meaning to experiences or anticipations of experiences. The meanings given to experiences are dynamic and can change in the light of further information which offers a different view of the situation.

This process is a human process and develops in childhood. From infancy the individual is building up information about the world and then giving meaning to the various aspects of it. There seem to be several levels to this, which overlap each other, so that an increasingly sophisticated and abstract interpretation of things overlays the more simplistic concrete representations. However, the more simplistic representations are still there and can be experienced as part of or instead of the more abstract ones, under stress. Many of the cognitive approaches to treatments or ways of helping people cope with pain are based on insights into these phenomena (see Chapter 8).

Chapter 6

Social and cultural aspects of pain

Pain passes – beauty remains.

Renoir

Introduction

This chapter follows the previous one very closely. Many of the points there were dependent on or related to interactions and relationships with others. Important significant others are, of course, family, parents in particular, and spouses. Friendship groups, neighbourhood groups, work groups are other examples of influential others who can affect the way we see the world and the place, role and behaviour of ourselves and others in it.

Social factors can influence the pain experience itself, not only the kind or bearability of the pain, but the way in which it is expressed. However, and as importantly, the pain can have an impact on others, through our relationships with them, particularly those very close to us.

We have referred, somewhat briefly, to some of the ways in which cognitive processes develop to enable us to make sense of our world. The influence of parents on the developing concepts and schemata for example have been considered, including the way children can imitate or copy the behaviour of others, most importantly parents or teachers. In particular we considered the role of communication in the exchange of ideas, information, values and beliefs in familial, social and societal situations.

In the previous chapter the emphasis was on the cognitive processes themselves and the social factors were examples of the ways that they may be influenced to develop in the way that they do. In this chapter we shall be concentrating more on the social factors themselves.

This chapter is divided into the following sections. First there will be some examples of the experiences of the social and cultural influences on pain and of pain on relationships. This will be followed by a consideration of the processes involved in creating these experiences, informed by research findings. Next there will be a discussion of the influence of pain on social relationships, including the family and in particular the spouse or partner. In each of these sections we will be considering aspects relating to both the acute and chronic pain situations. However, it is from the chronic pain situation that there is most influence on the family and other social relationships. Then we shall consider some of the socio-economic implications of the pain experience, particularly chronic pain, and finally we shall look at cultural aspects of the pain experience.

The patient's experiences

Communication

In the acute pain situation the patient will be aware of ways of behaving when in pain. These will be communicated to the individual from childhood when parents would provide examples of expected behaviour, or would encourage or punish particular behaviours. Thus the person experiencing pain will learn either not to make too much fuss or to cry out and demand attention (Zborowski 1952; Gaffney and Dunne 1987). The ability to cope with the pain, the bearability of the pain, will depend on whether or not the behaviour is acceptable and the individual feels that he or she is playing their role properly as expected. If so then attention would be given and the pain dealt with as effectively as possible, psychological support and comfort will be given as well as physical treatment.

The question of the expression of pain or pain-related behaviour is particularly important in the social setting. There are social or even familial norms to be met, or adhered to. These will determine whether or not the person in pain will feel able to cry out for example, or to complain. This can be very important in childhood and parental influences can be very strong, particularly with the older child. With younger children there may be a more idiosyncratic pattern of behaviour, with the child perhaps being quiet and withdrawn, but showing signs of strain or shock. Alternatively, there may be much noise and movement, and yet the apparent stimulation may seem the same. Parents are very good guides as to what particular kinds of behaviour might mean. They can help to determine what if anything is wrong. Indeed they may report that the child just feels different from how they usually feel when they hold them, or behaves differently, without being able to put their finger on the cause exactly. This was demonstrated in an unpublished study by the author. This involved interviews with parents and professionals about indicators of pain in young children. Twenty-one members of staff were interviewed and thirty parents, mainly mothers. Being different for one child may mean crying and being restless; for another it may mean being quiet and withdrawn, or clinging and cuddling.

In the chronic pain situation, the meaning of the pain for the sufferer has particular relevance to the social setting. In terms of pain behaviour, the sufferer will be entered into particular relationships with professionals, and his or her behaviour will reflect the patient's perception of these relationships and roles (Strauss *et al.* 1963; Goffman 1974, and for a critique, Brooking 1986). This perception of the relationships and roles can influence the bearability of the pain and even its perceived intensity.

Emotional and cognitive aspects

The emotional reaction to the pain can be influenced by the relationships with others. Feelings of uncertainty and anxiety can be increased or decreased by the actions or communications of others (Hayward 1975; Johnson *et al.* 1991). Similarly feelings of confidence in the future, of hope, of being brave and coping can be generated by others in the information that they give and so help to prevent depressive feelings arising (Roy 1992). Sometimes the patient may feel very unsure of him or herself, not understanding what they should or could do for themselves. If they naturally like being in control and looking after themselves, then having this control taken away, being put into a more passive role and/or lacking information can be very distressing and affect the perception of the pain (Affleck *et al.* 1987).

If we refer back to the experiences described in the chapters on the motivational and emotional, and the cognitive-evaluative, aspects of pain then we can see that all of these have the potential to be influenced by the social aspects. Many of these will be stored as memories, and the person in pain may not be immediately aware of the source of the influences. They may go back to childhood, or be associated with growing up with or living amongst a particular group of people. The neighbourhood groups, the religious groups, the cultural groups, with whom the person in pain is associated, however loosely, will each have norms and expectations (Helman 1994).

Group influences on the pain experience

These norms and expectations will be communicated to the individual in a variety of ways, through school or church, for example. Important or popular people will set an example which may be communicated via the media. In plays, documentaries and TV series, examples will be given of pain-related behaviour. The individual watching these will be able to imitate the behaviour of those people or characters he or she admires or wishes to emulate. This may be a conscious act with the person trying to act in a particular way to live up to some ideal. This links in with the discussion in Chapter 4 on the satisfaction of needs and in particular those of self-actualisation.

The person in pain will have been receiving this information throughout his or her life, or during membership of a particular group, almost without being aware of it. The concepts and schemata created through cognitive processes, linked to the emotional centres, will incorporate these subtle influences. As well as influences from the past and recent times, there will of course be influences from the present, and there is great potential for influence from social sources and significant others. These might of course include professionals who can play an important role in the management of the pain experience.

Influence of pain on social relationships

Another major aspect of the link between pain and social factors is the influence of the person's pain on others with whom the person has relationships or with whom he or she is associated. Immediate effects will be on the individual's family and those close to him or her (Roy 1992). With children this will be the parents, and with older people, the spouse or partner. Others, members of the various groups to which the person belongs, such as neighbourhood groups and work groups, will also be affected.

The pain will affect such people through the roles that are played by the person within these groups or with the particular people. The roles and relationships may have to be changed, such as with a husband or wife, or of an adult with an elderly parent. A relationship of dependency may change in respect to the degree of disability or incapacity created by the chronic pain. A child may be more dependent on a parent; a parent may become dependent on an older child; an older person may be dependent on an adult son or daughter; and an adult son or daughter may become dependent again on an older parent. There will be emotional aspects to these changes also, with psychological distress, depression, and even anger and hostility being experienced or expressed.

Work relationships and other social, community relationships may also be affected in terms of the roles held or the parts played in the various activities associated with these groups. Roy (1985) has given some excellent case examples of the social implications of chronic pain. These clearly and often dramatically illustrate these influences of the pain experience on social and interpersonal relationships. For example, there may be an effect on sexual relationships with a partner as the person in pain does not feel up to it or the partner does not wish to cause further pain. There may be a strong sense of loss associated with the chronic pain situation or of guilt leading to a depressive response which may interfere with sexual activity. The person may become shy and withdrawn because of the limitations caused by the pain and feel unworthy of such a physical relationship.

Alternatively the person with the pain may use it to opt out of unwelcome social responsibilities or engagements. The pain may cause stress which itself can cause other conflicts or interpersonal difficulties to come to the surface and become unmanageable. There may be anger, or a sense of demoralisation which may destroy existing but shaky relationships. Even if the incapacity caused by the pain is not sufficient to prevent the person from doing his or her job, the pain may cause relationships at work to deteriorate as the emotional burden is perhaps shared with colleagues. If there is a loss of occupation then the relationships in the home will be influenced as perhaps there has to be a change of roles with the wife becoming the major wage earner and the husband taking on more of the home making or child-rearing role. With a single person there may be a return of dependency on an elderly parent, or a relative, or even a neighbour. There may be the situation of a person in their eighties with their own health problems having to support a person in their fifties with incapacitating chronic pain.

Conclusion

The person with these effects on their social relationships will also be subject to feelings of responsibility, anxiety and depression at causing this burden on others. This reciprocal relationship between social factors and pain may make the situation worse, increasing the emotional aspects of the situation. There may be a reciprocal feeling of guilt or worthlessness as these roles change. Loss of employment and subsequent financial worries, a failure to play an important role in the local community may also lead to isolation and withdrawal with associated distress. Motivation to start or continue with treatments may be affected by these social implications of chronic pain (Roy 1992).

In the following section we shall consider the processes and mechanisms that bring about these experiences of the person in pain, from a social and cultural perspective. We shall be demonstrating links with the previous chapters as these social factors influence the cognitive-evaluative and the emotional and the sensory-discriminative process of the experience of pain. This is a most important area of the study of the pain experience and leads to many kinds of psycho-social methods of treatment as complements to or alternatives to pharmacological and physical ones. Nevertheless it does relate to those also, as the influence can involve those aspects of the pain experience.

Social influences on the pain experience

When we attempt to study the different effects of social factors on pain as experienced by the sufferer we find that we can consider them under four main headings: social learning theory; role relationships; socio-economic aspects; and culture. The latter also in many ways embraces the other three as will be seen when we come to that section. Social learning theory underpins and attempts to explain role expectations as well as the influence of cultural factors (Bandura 1977). All four are of course influences on the cognitive and evaluative processes that are involved in the experience of pain. The cognitive-evaluative aspects are also closely related to the emotional and motivational aspects which can be influenced by social and cultural expectations. There is also some evidence that the sensory-discriminative aspects of pain are influenced by social and cultural influences.

In the following sections therefore we shall be considering the psycho-social principles behind the processes that bring about these influences and some research into the experience of pain that supports them.

Social learning theory

When we consider the development of concepts and schemata which enable us to create a mental model of the world and our relationships within it, an important point made was that of Vygotsky's communication model of cognitive development and processes (1986). In this model he emphasised the role of communication in providing information which would then be processed to produce the developing concepts and schemata, mental models stored in our memories. Communication of course implies other people with whom to communicate.

Some of the concepts are developed by the individual interacting with other aspects of his or her environment. However, much of the time is spent with other people and hence the importance of social communication. The communication may be through the media of course. Nevertheless it originates with other people as writers, teachers, radio or television presenters or actors (see National Institute of Mental Health 1982; Clifford *et al.* 1995). Much communication is non-verbal, in that we observe others undergoing experiences, trying out things, demonstrating things and we learn from that form of communication too.

The learning thus is derived from a variety of different interactions with members of different groups (Moscovici 1988). This leads to comparisons of self with others, their behaviour attitudes and values (Festinger 1954), particularly with relevant others, for example from the peer group or particular significant others (Sanders 1982). Sartorious (1991) has identified three levels of social comparison: individual, a comparison with ideal self; interpersonal, a comparison with relevant social groups; and socio-cultural, a comparison with societal expectations, medical opinion and the media (see Skevington 1995).

These comparisons also lead to the development of one's social identity (Tajfel 1978), but can be downward as well (Wills 1991). In a small-scale phenomenological study, Osborn and Smith (1998) found the use of comparisons with others as well as with themselves in the past as being important for those experiencing pain to make sense of the experience. However, the results of these comparisons could have both positive and negative effects. In effect these comparisons lead to 'a structured system of beliefs that is widely shared with others and is constantly changing through discussion' (Skevington 1995, p. 123).

Social learning theory draws also on behavioural learning theory and in particular the principle of reinforcement. Bandura (1967) describes how children copy the behaviour of adults, especially if the adult is rewarded in some way. However, there is no need for the child to be rewarded themselves for the behaviour to be repeated and for learning to occur. Penner and Rioux (1995) have identified empathic behaviour in adults which they learnt through modelling as children. Such vicarious conditioning is thought to be behind much social learning and the mechanism behind cultural influences also. Koutantji et al. (1998) have reported a study of students and their current pain experiences. The students reported the use of models with the female students reporting a greater use of models for pain behaviour, which suggests a gender difference in awareness of pain in others.

Fordyce (1976) has considered specifically the role of reinforcement in pain behaviour, and this has been taken further by Turk and Flor (1987) who identified different types of reinforcement (see above).

Social learning theory (Bandura 1977) builds on the work of many others to provide a description and an explanation of this process of learning how to behave and how to value things. Others have arrived at similar conclusions from different sources (see, for example, Kelly (1955, 1991) and his study of role relationships, significant others and personal constructs). This approach benefited also from the insights of such writers as Mead (1934) and Schutz (1960). They attempted to demonstrate the reliance we all have on others in coping with the vicissitudes of everyday life.

Mead was concerned with the ideas of self, the 'me' and the 'I', and he felt that these were both linked to our relationships with others, in particular our 'significant others'. Kelly (1955, 1991) argued that we each approach the world as experimenters, testing out hypotheses and from the results, building a view of how to deal effectively with it. This includes other people and, indeed, Kelly's main concern was with our relationships with other people and how we construe them. By this is meant our explanation and expectation as to how they are likely to behave, and in particular how they will behave towards us. The way we construe ourselves is related to these constructs about the others. Our picture of ourselves and the way we would expect to behave is very much related to the way we expect others to behave and particularly with respect towards us, or in situations similar to ours.

By construing we develop constructs which describe or explain or predict our relationships with others and their relationships with us. We also construe situations, events and aspects of our lives other than people, and we construe other people in relation to these events in our lives or in similar situations. These constructs or descriptions, explanations, predictions, indicate how we have seen other people behaving in particular situations, or how we would expect them to behave based on other kinds of experience and information about them construed on different occasions. If their behaviour is successful, or has been in the past, then that will be built into our construct system, and thus their usefulness to us or otherwise as being able to play a role for us is determined.

Kelly (1955, 1991) built this model into a successful therapeutic process to help people cope with their relationships. Large and Strong (1997) have used Repertory Grid Technique to explore the meaning of coping for chronic pain patients, who found it a necessary evil (see Beail (1985) for examples including education and management).

Roles and pain behaviour

We all play a variety of roles in the various aspects of our lives. Each of these is in relation to a particular group of people – the role set – who are themselves playing particular roles in relation to the activities or purpose of the group. The roles may have a wider meaning and reflect expectations not only for the particular group but for the wider society and culture within which the group functions (see Turner 1962; Krech *et al.* 1971).

Expectations are the behaviours (including attitudes and values expressed) that should be carried out by the person in a particular role. They are 'sent' by the others in the group, and by the wider society. To be a member of a group means accepting the role and the associated behaviours, provided that there is a clear understanding by the role player of the expectations for that role. Then the person can fit in with that particular group and the wider society. If there is role ambiguity caused by lack of information, or understanding of the expected behaviour, attitudes or values of a particular role, then this can cause difficulties and the person may have a problem fitting in or being accepted by the other members of the group. It may lead to rejection from the group or even from the wider society.

A person may have a role in one group and another in a different group. If the expectations for these two roles are incompatible then this can lead to role conflict, and be a source of stress to the individual as well as leading to failure to perform either or both of the roles properly.

Another form of role conflict can occur when there are different views or interpretations of expectations within a group for a particular role. This also may lead to difficulty in or a failure to perform satisfactorily in the role. There even may be different assessments by members of the group as to the appropriateness of the behaviour. The individual may feel that they are behaving as expected and yet other members may feel the behaviour is not appropriate. This may happen if there are expectations from a wider social group or culture which are influencing the individual and to which he or she is responding, but of which the other members of the group are not aware or misunderstand.

Health-related roles

There are many groups in which the behavioural expectations may change or differ. The person in pain has to be aware of the expected behaviour for a person in pain in any particular group, such as a family group, a work group, a health-care group. This can be difficult, because, unless he or she has had much previous experience of pain, it may be an unfamiliar role. The social learning that has occurred about pain behaviour, gained for example by the person in real life or from the media, will give some preparation. The media, in particular television, can be very influential in the social learning process (National Institute of Mental Health 1982; Clifford *et al.* 1995).

There will also have been learning from parents and others as to how to behave when in pain (Gaffney and Dunne 1987). This will be incorporated into the person's own expectations as to how to behave when in pain, the expectations which will inform his or her general behaviour unless there are any other clearly expressed expectations from any other source.

There are generally accepted, socially constructed expectations of the role of a sick person. This was described by Parsons (1951), and these expectations reflect the values and beliefs of the particular society. These expectations are supposed to be accepted by all members of the society and of the groups within it. Even decisions about what is an acceptable illness, the course of that illness and the behaviour expected of someone suffering from that illness are socially constructed (Blaxter and Paterson 1982; Calman and Johnson 1985; Armstrong 1983). These definitions and expectations may vary from society to society and we shall consider this again when considering cultural aspects of pain.

Some of the definitions of illness and expectations of sick role behaviour are put out (sent) by the health-care professionals, and by doctors in particular (Kennedy 1981). If the person in pain is not aware of these expectations or definitions then they may find it difficult to act in an acceptable way, or if they are aware of them, in a way that satisfies their own expectations of how they feel they should, or would like to, act. The medical, health-care sick role can have expectations of a relatively passive patient who is 'treated' or 'cared for' in a way determined by the health-care team. This has led to attempts to classify patients into different types (Duff and Hollingshead 1968), or the identification of 'good' and 'bad' patients (Stockwell 1972; Kelly and May 1982; Davis 1984c). This can lead to labelling of patients as deviants (Evers 1981). They have even be given derogatory labels, such as 'the usual rubbish' (Jeffrey 1979).

Some of these labelling functions are related to beliefs about the origin of disease, the definition of disease (signs and symptoms) (Pilowski 1990; Pilowski and Katsikitis 1994), and are based on judgements by the professionals (Leavitt 1985). There are strong arguments against this approach to medicalise illness (see Szasz 1973; Illich 1976; Kleinman 1988) and this will be considered further in the section on cultural aspects of pain.

More recently there have been attempts to accept the individuality of the patient, particularly in nursing, in terms of their own interpretations and expectations. Also there have been attempts to involve them in a more active role, as expressed in recent writings on models of nursing (e.g. Orem 1995; King 1981; Leininger 1991; Roper *et al.* 1990; Roy 1996; and see McKenna 1997 for a critique).

Other recent approaches include that of partnerships between professionals and the client (e.g. Salvage 1985). However, the person in pain, as part of the health-care group, will have their own expectations of expert help, either a passive or an active role, and a need for information. If these are not met then there will be conflict and role stress.

Although Parsons (1951) articulated the idea of the sick role as being an expectation of the hospital medical world of that time and it was to a certain extent supported by Strauss *et al.* (1963) as a negotiated order of roles (including those of doctor and nurse and other positions within the hierarchy) (see also Merton 1957; Goffman 1974), there have been criticisms of this (Fitton and Ascherson 1979; Brooking 1986). In many ways this negotiated order reflected aspects of power, such as those described by French and Raven (1968) (see Box 6.1).

This need to tightly structure roles and relationships in the health-care setting is related to ideas of control (Fagerhaugh and Strauss 1977), particularly the control of information (Bond 1978), and the management of uncertainty and unpredictability. This has been seen as particularly important in the clinical areas, and the

---

Box 6.1   Aspects of power

Reward	The ability to offer others, for example, money, promotion, preference or other kinds of reward
Coercion	The ability to force others, perhaps through threats of punishment or withdrawal of favours
Legitimate authority	Power conferred by some higher authority, as in being placed in a particular position in an organisation, and having control of access and information for example
Expert	Power derived from expert knowledge known only to a select few
Referent	Being respected and admired, charisma
	(French and Raven 1968)

functional management of organisations (Davies 1983; Rosenthal *et al.*
1980). Another aspect has been the routinisation of care practices,
negating individual needs in an attempt to cope with uncertainty,
and the emotional demands on staff of caring for people in pain, or
approaching death (Bond 1978).

Impact of pain on role

There are two main effects on role brought about by chronic pain.
The main effects are of course in relation to those closest to the
person in pain, and those for whom he or she plays an important
role or spends a lot of time. These are effects on family structure
and function, and effects on employment. The closest relationships
are usually with the family (Roy 1992). However, some people can
become very close to work mates or colleagues, as much time is
spent with them and if working in stressful conditions, the degree of
interdependence can be very great and, in particular, involve
emotional dependence. This is often experienced at the time of
retirement when the 'loss' of work and the relationships with mates
or colleagues can be quite severe. If the loss is due to leaving work
for reasons of illness and in particular chronic pain, then the fact
that the pain has caused this loss can influence the attitude towards
the pain. A sense of isolation can be very detrimental in the chronic
pain situation, and Rose (1994) has argued for the careful assessment of this aspect. This is related to sensory restriction caused by a
change in social relations or work activity which can also be influential (Schofield and Davis 1998), although on-going work indicates
that sensory stimulation (as in a Snoezelen facility) might be of
benefit here.

The family

As far as the family is concerned it is the relationship with the
spouse that is most affected although the whole family can be affected
if there are substantial changes to the financial status of the family
group. Research into the effects of chronic pain on the family has
used models of normal family function for comparison. For example,
the McMaster Model of Family Functioning has been used by Roy
(1988). This model has six factors that are compared between the
various groups: problem solving; communication; roles; affective
responsiveness; affective involvement; and behavioural control.

Looking at the effect of chronic pain on families Roy (1988) found a great deal of disturbance. For each of the factors more than 50 per cent of the families showed disruption and breakdown of roles and relationships. This was a very small sample but did involve intensive interviews.

In further studies of larger groups, and using other models, such as the Family Adaptability and Cohesion Evaluation Scale (Olson *et al.*1984), Roy and Thomas (1989) found the families to be operating at the 'chaotic' level of functioning. This study concentrated in particular on the relationship of the couples, and focused on roles; rules; decision making; discipline; and leadership. The spouses tended to be performing at a more effective level, although they were affected themselves. Interestingly there was no difference between short-term pain and long-term pain situations, suggesting that the effects happen early. Simmonds *et al.* (1998) argue that the impact of the chronic pain on the family is related to their health beliefs and coping strategies as a family, as did Snelling (1994). This would also reflect societal and cultural influences. Keefe *et al.* (1998) also found that pain-coping strategies influenced self-ratings of self-efficacy of sufferers and spouses. Roy (1992) notes with concern the lack of research into the effects of chronic pain on the children in these dysfunctional families, and refers to a similar comment by Flor *et al.* (1987). This is obviously an area warranting research.

Pain and sexual relationships

There is evidence that sexual abuse has a link with later pain experiences, particularly with respect to pelvic and gastro-intestinal pain. This is with relation to self-reported sexual abuse. The actual incidence of abuse is difficult to estimate and perhaps is irrelevant. Repeated studies have demonstrated this link as reviewed by Thomas (1997), who related it back to the work of Engel (1959), and by Linton (1997). Linton *et al.* (1996) confirmed this link, in particular with musculo-skeletal pain, and also demonstrated that with females, physical abuse increased the risk of pronounced pain by five-fold and sexual abuse increased it by four-fold (Linton 1997). Goldberg *et al.* (1999) found significant relationships between childhood abuse and later alcoholism, drug addiction and chronic pain. They argue that from their study, childhood abuse is a wider phenomenon than just physical and sexual abuse, and involves whole family dysfunction.

A major aspect of the effect on the couples involves the sexual relationship. Many studies have reported evidence of sexual dysfunction (Maruta and Osborne 1978; Flor *et al.* 1987; Roy 1988). Roy (1989) suggests that there might be a pre-morbid history of sexual problems, depression or other interpersonal reasons for these problems (see also Walker *et al.* 1990); however, in many cases the pain itself does seem to be the cause (see Roy (1992) for a review of this aspect of chronic pain). However, Monga *et al.* (1998) argue that it is the level of disability and psychological distress including depression that influences the sexual dysfunction rather than the pain itself.

Depression in the spouse is a not uncommon outcome (Shanfield *et al.* 1979; Flor *et al.* 1987). This often reflects a change in their role and the development of role conflicts (Hudgens 1979; Rowat and Knafl 1985). The spouse, if not already, frequently has to become the main wage earner, and this often applies to the wife if the husband is the sufferer. Similarly a change of role from the wage earner to include home maker as well is often a major strain for the husband, if the person in pain is the wife. Negative responses from the spouse seem to have different effects depending on gender, with both emotions and pain severity being affected. The complicated and variable nature of these associations as demonstrated by Burns *et al.* (1996) confirms the importance of taking an individualistic approach in the assessment of the pain experience.

Work and employment

If the sufferer is in pain but continuing to work there can be an effect on the relationships with co-workers. This may reflect an inability to carry out the full work role, increasing the burden of others. This may lead to complaints and the sufferer being picked on or excluded from friendship groups (Roy 1992). They may be accused of malingering, of trying to escape from unpleasant duties or responsibilities, although there is little hard evidence in support of malingering as an important aspect of chronic pain (Skevington 1995). Then the onus is on the sufferer to confirm the existence of pain with evidence other than just their word. There does seem to be little evidence that people in pain exaggerate it in order to support their claim, or indeed report higher levels of pain or disability

(Mendelson 1984, 1986). Sheikh (1987) found that a history of occupational injury appears to have an adverse effect on return to work.

There is the complication of disability to consider as well as the pain, for injury-related pain may also involve some form of physical or mental damage (Follick *et al.* 1984; Sanders 1983). However, Leavitt and Sweet (1986), following a survey, have estimated that 3 per cent of chronic pain sufferers are malingering. Trief and Stein (1985) have found that there are some personality differences between those who make claims and those who do not. The former tend to be more likely to disclose troubles and intimate details about themselves. Gallagher *et al.* (1989), commenting on the over-emphasis on physical assessment of disability and a failure to consider psychological and social aspects, have argued that applying for compensation was not an indication of a desire to avoid work.

Achievement of financial compensation does not seem to improve the rate of return to work or to reduce the reports of high levels of pain (Tunks 1990). However, Becker *et al.* (1998) argue that gaining a disability pension did lead to improvement in pain and social functioning. They suggested that many of the problems of people with chronic pain are related to socio-economic factors. Thus the evidence for malingering or of exaggeration of symptoms does seem to be inconclusive although the number of claims for compensation is a major financial problem at a national level. Different countries have developed a variety of schemes to manage compensation and benefit systems. However, this does make it difficult to compare the different systems, as the statistical models used to keep account of the phenomenon vary so much (Skevington 1995).

Socio-economic aspects of pain

When one considers the number of people in chronic pain, the socio-economic effects do not only involve the cost of compensation and benefit. There is also the lost productivity, in terms of work; or of family support of work in terms of the effect on the family of the pain (Latham and Davis 1994). Estimates of the incidence of chronic pain in the USA for example include 23 million suffering from back ache and 24 million suffering from headache (Brena and Chapman 1983; Escobar 1985). Bonica (1974) estimated nearly 35 per cent of Americans were affected by pain. Schmitt (1985), estimated that 80 per cent of visits to physicians were for low back pain. Costs as high as $50 billion have been suggested (Schmitt 1985; Turk *et al.*

1983), and that 5 million Americans were pain-related beneficiaries of Social Security (Escobar 1985).

It has been suggested that up to 45 million working days are lost because of back pain each year with treatment for this condition costing approximately £193 million each year (Rigge 1990; and more recently confirmed by Waddell 1996). Following a recent review of the literature on prevalence of chronic benign pain, Verhaak *et al.* (1998) demonstrate a wide range of prevalence rates, which could not be explained by research methods nor definition of chronic pain. They tentatively suggest a prevalence of chronic pain of 10 per cent. They suggest also that the effects of the pain in terms of disability, loss of work, premature incapacity or unnecessary medical treatment as being more important than trying to find accurate estimates of the number of patients experiencing pain each day.

Reid *et al.* (1997) have reviewed several studies and estimate that some 95 per cent of people suffering from back pain return to work within 6–12 weeks. It would seem that relatively few of the chronic pain sufferers account for the majority of the costs, in terms of health-related costs and disability and compensation costs. The health-care costs are only a small proportion of the total costs (e.g. van Tulder *et al.* (1995) in the Netherlands, and the National Board of Health and Welfare in Sweden (1987)). In spite of this, that small proportion does not seem to be being well spent according to Linton (1998) who has reviewed the current situation. He argues for programmes of care that incorporate a multi-dimensional view of the problem. In particular it is suggested that the psycho-social aspects of the problem are emphasised, based on a thorough, 'low-tech', examination (p.166), plus a detailed feedback to the person in pain, and the development of a programme which is based on self-care. Also he argues for the reduction of anxiety, detailed recommendations about activities and graded exercises, and finally the non-medicalisation of the pain situation.

Quality of life

Many of the effects of chronic pain described above in fact relate to the quality of life of people in pain. This has been a major area of concern recently and many different health-care problems have been studied as to their effect on quality of life. One of the problems is that of definition. There have been many attempts, for example that of Williams (1985), who described a quality-adjusted life year as a measure of impact on life. Thus there might be a long life span predicted with a certain problem, but the crucial aspect according to Williams was the quality of those life years. Thus a long life, but with much reduced quality, might not be as good as a shorter life span, but with a much higher level of quality.

Another approach was that of Benner (1985) who discussed the quality of being in an attempt to incorporate more abstract aspects of life, and Revicky (1989) considered the issue of a health-related quality of life. A review of models by Meerburg (1993) with a concept analysis identified the following definition: a feeling of overall satisfaction as determined by the individual who is mentally alert. The person must be seen as living in conditions that are adequate and meeting basic needs.

There is a problem here with the interpretation of the term 'mentally alert'. Tarter *et al.* (1988) identified possession of behavioural and cognitive abilities; emotional well-being; and ability to perform domestic, vocational and social roles as comprising mental alertness. The importance of leisure was discussed by Tomlinson (1991) with social isolation seen very much as a negative factor (Rigge 1990). With a Danish sample of chronic patients, Becker *et al.* (1997) demonstrated a very poor quality of life for these patients, on a variety of dimensions, including sleep, anxiety and depression and general psychological and social well-being.

Skevington (1995) has reviewed this area and comments that there has been an emphasis on the development of instruments to measure the phenomenon of quality of life, without the development of a theoretical model to inform that development. Black (1992) has developed a model of chronic pain, however, and argues that the best measurement of quality of life in relation to pain is the view of the sufferer him or herself; this is supported by Hunt and McKenna (1992). Skevington (1998) has explored this area further using the WHOQOL instrument developed by the WHOQOL group, an international group set up by the WHO to develop such an instrument. Skevington's study attempted to use the instrument with pain patients. Pain and discomfort is one of the aspects of quality of life included in the instrument. Evidence of reliability and validity was found to support the use of the instrument with people in pain. With respect to the quality of life of people in pain the study found that a longer duration of pain was associated with increasingly poor quality of life and this was exacerbated by intense emotional aspects of the pain experience.

Cultural aspects of pain

We have been looking at the various groups and relationships that individuals belong to and with whom they live and work and have their friendships. All these groups and relationships are set in a larger society and that larger society itself has influence, on the groups, the families and the individual. By sharing information, beliefs and strategies for coping we all benefit.

In this final section to this chapter we shall consider some of the ways in which people can be influenced by their culture, and with special reference to the effect that influence can have on the pain experience. In particular we shall look at what we mean by the term culture; how it affects health and illness behaviour; and finally how it affects pain. This section is based on a more substantive review published elsewhere (Davis 1998).

What is culture?

It has been variously defined as guidelines (Helman 1994); systems of shared ideas, concepts, rules (Keesing 1981); and values, beliefs, norms and lifeways (Leininger 1991). The purpose of these guidelines, lifeways and rules is to help people belonging to a society to cope with the challenges affecting that society. In particular they help them to behave in relation to other people as well as the environment and supernatural aspects. They help in decision making and the particular meaning to be put on events or experiences.

In order to be part of a culture one has to accept these guidelines, rules and lifeways. There is a sense of 'we' and 'they', and of a common fate, with a tendency to interact more among themselves than with others, and the term ethnic group is often applied (Smooha 1985). The degree of identification with the cultural or ethnic group by an individual will determine the degree to which he or she will be influenced by the rules, lifeways and guidelines. This can be difficult when there is one ethnic group living as a sub-group within a larger society and with a requirement to live up to the guidelines, rules and lifeways of both groups. In the modern western world this frequently occurs, particularly in the UK and the USA. Some of the research to be discussed below reflects this.

Culture, health and illness behaviour

Kleinman *et al.* (1978) have argued that illness behaviour is very much influenced by societal and cultural norms. This can be complicated particularly with reference to sub-cultures and the individual can respond to western medical models and practices, the formal medical model of the home culture, or the models offered in folk or traditional medicine associated with the home culture (Kleinman *et al.* 1978). Models illustrating the bio-psycho-social aspects of disease have been offered by the WHO (1980), Kleinman (1988), and Helman (1994). The relationships between professional and lay involvement in the determination of health and illness is demonstrated in Box 6.2.

These levels or aspects reflect very much the approach taken in our analysis and discussion of the pain experience so far, with the sensory-discriminative, cognitive-evaluative, motivational-emotional, and socio-cultural aspects. A failure on the part of a practitioner to be sensitive and responsive to the illness and sickness aspects of the disease and the patient's experience will affect any therapeutic relationship that might be developing, and perhaps ultimately the patient's response to or compliance with any therapy.

In many cultures there are two languages relating to health and illness: the medical language and the folk or lay language (Helman

---

Box 6.2   The bio-psycho-social aspects of disease

- **Disease** is the diagnosis of a medical practitioner with associated signs and treatments (often physiological) – the practitioner's view.
- **Illness or impairment** is the experience of the patient with various symptoms and meanings to those symptoms (often physiological and experiential) – the patient's view.
- **Sickness as disability** is the impact of the disease or illness on the physical or mental functioning of the patient (often physiological, psychological and social) – the social view.
- **Sickness as handicap** is the impact of the disease and illness suffered by the individual, on the family, or work situation (often physiological, psychological and social) – the societal view.

1994). They may reflect different understandings of disease and illness and treatment. Folk or lay perceptions frequently reflect more cultural values. The ways in which ill-health is reported will reflect these lay, cultural factors. Thus we may find that men and women present their symptoms differently; that the family may be more or less involved; there may be more or less emotional expression of the situation; supernatural influences may be reported.

Culture and pain

There does seem to be evidence that people from different cultures experience and express pain in different ways. However, there does not seem to be any evidence that people from different cultures have a different sensory experience of pain. Melzack and Wall (1996) suggest three levels or kinds of potential cultural influence. The first, the sensory level, they argue, is the same for all people and they refer to the work of Sternbach and Tursky (1965); the second is the pain perception threshold. They refer to the work of Hardy *et al.* (1952) comparing Mediterranean and northern Europeans, and Clark and Clark (1980) comparing Nepalese and westerners. There is however limited research in this area. The third level is that of pain tolerance threshold. They refer to the work of Zborowski (1952); Lambert *et al.* (1960); Woodrow *et al.* (1972); and Clark and Clark (1980).

However, there also does seem to be evidence of different ways of expressing pain, which may have influenced these findings. This often involves the emotional and cognitive-evaluative aspects of the pain. Zborowski (1952) for example reported different levels of emotional expression, although there are criticisms of this study in that different cultures were amalgamated into larger groups for the analysis. Fabrega and Tyma (1976) demonstrated linguistic and semantic differences between cultures. Attempts to develop different language versions of the McGill Pain Questionnaire have demonstrated the different number and kinds of words for pain in other languages (see Melzack and Katz (1992) for a review of the different versions). The different versions have been generated using native speakers to obtain culturally valid verbalisations of the pain experience (Thomas (1997) has discussed this issue with particular reference to assessment; see also Chapter 9). There is much potential for research into the cognitive processes involved in the perception of pain, using comparisons of the kinds of words and linguistic structures used by people from different cultures and languages to explore the semantic aspects of the experience.

Comparing different cultures, Robinson (1990) identified three main types of expression of pain: the tragic, the sad, and the heroic. Differences in expression of pain in children have also been reported (Zborowski 1952; Perrin and Gerrity 1982; Gaffney and Dunne 1987). These results demonstrate the role of parents in the development of culturally determined responses. Others have also demonstrated the development of responses to pain in children, echoing the levels of cognitive development (Savendra *et al*. 1982; Brewster 1982). These seem to follow the Piagetian model of levels of development and the increasingly less concrete and more abstract formulations, as development proceeds (see Chapter 5).

Two studies have shown different responses to pain between Mexican Americans and Anglo-Americans. In Kosko and Flaskerud (1987) the main difference was between the utilisation of folk models of health and illness regarding chest pain. With the same cultural groups but concentrating on women, Calvillo and Flaskerud (1993) showed no difference between the pain responses of the two groups, as measured by the McGill Pain Questionnaire, medication and vital signs. However, nurses rated the pain experienced by the two groups differently and as being less severe than as assessed by the patients themselves. These latter findings will be discussed in more detail in the chapter on the management of pain. Thus these two studies suggest that culture influences the meaning of the pain more than its intensity. There were educational and social status differences between the groups which might also reflect the different meanings.

Although we see ourselves as individuals, with our own way of looking at and responding to our environment, and although we, as nurses, or health-care professionals, try to treat our patients and people in our care as individuals, we must also be aware that both we and they are the product of a variation of influences from social interactions. These make up the particular persona presented by each individual. Our assessments, our plans of care and our treatments must bear in mind that, although the pain belongs to the sufferer, and its presence, meaning and intensity are as declared by the individual, the person in pain is a member of a family, playing roles in a health-care system, in a work and a social and cultural environment. The pain experience is very much influenced by and is influencing these factors.

Conclusion

Thus it does seem that there is some influence from culture on the pain experience and its expression. The meaning of the pain, the language and emotional aspects of its expression are all vulnerable to such influence. However, it does also seem that individuals vary in the extent to which they are influenced by the culture in which they live, depending on the degree of their integration into or acceptance of its values, rules and guidelines. There is also evidence that some of these influences occur in childhood when the behaviours and meanings are acquired.

There is obviously a link with the social aspects of pain as discussed in the previous section, where social learning was considered. Also the way in which the meanings and behaviours, and how to deal with them, are added to the developing set of concepts and schemata of life were considered in the previous chapter. Many of these cultural influences affect the emotional expression of the pain and relate to the issues discussed in Chapter 4, looking at emotion and motivation. The effects of culture on the individual's tolerance of pain relate very closely to the issues and processes described and discussed in the earlier chapter on sensory-discriminative aspects of pain.

Thus in this part of the book we have demonstrated a closely integrated bio-psycho-socio-cultural system which offers a great deal of insight into the experience of pain. It enables the practitioner or carer to have a greater awareness of what is happening to the person in pain and from that to be able to play a more insightful, meaningful and hopefully more effective role in the management of the pain.

The information provided by access to this inside story of the pain experience is of vital importance if the assessment of the pain is to offer any meaningful information on which to base an effective plan of care. This information and understanding is also important regarding the choice of therapeutic intervention, the role of the person in pain in the decision-making process and in any therapy that might be provided or offered.

Our approach to the next part of the book will be based on this inside story. As we consider and discuss the types of therapeutic intervention; aspects of the assessment of pain; and the management issues, it will be important to bear in mind, and reference will be made back to, the issues considered and the evidence presented in the chapters in this part.

Part III

Interventions to help the person in pain

Chapter 7

Pharmacological and physical interventions

Pleasure is nothing else but the intermission of pain.

Selden

Introduction

The reason for exploring in some detail the mechanisms of pain and the experiences of those in pain is to help us to have a more effective approach to intervening with and helping those in pain. In other words the expectation is that the more our interventions are based on or related to the mechanisms described and discussed in the preceding chapters, the more successful they will be. This is where a full assessment of the experience is most important – this is dealt with in Chapter 9. The assessment must explore all those aspects of the experience that are amenable to some form of treatment or other. The various aspects of the experience described in Chapters 3, 4, 5 and 6 demonstrate the range of the potential need in the management of pain. In this and the next chapter the range of treatments available is explored so that when we come to the assessment of pain and the administration of interventions in Chapters 9 and 10 we can tie together the various aspects of the experience, the interventions available, and the care.

Two main types of intervention are presented in this and the following chapter. First those that relate to the biochemical and physiological mechanisms described above (mainly in Chapters 3 and 4). That is those related to the sensory-discriminative and the motivational and emotional aspects of pain. The main interventions here therefore are drugs and various physical interventions. The second type, to be considered in the next chapter, is psychological interventions which are concerned largely with the cognitive-evaluative, but also to a certain extent with the social and cultural aspects too. These involve enabling the person in pain to feel differently about the pain situation, to find ways of living with or thinking about the pain, as well as helping the social situations that can result from living with pain. There is some overlap however with some psychological interventions affecting the emotional-motivational aspects.

This chapter then is concerned with those interventions that involve bringing about changes in the biochemical mechanisms that facilitate the transmission of the noxious stimuli through the peripheral and central nervous systems to the brain and the experience of pain. There are also however drugs that facilitate the downward transmission of signals that interfere with the transmission of the noxious stimulus, closing the gate so to speak. These interventions involve the administration of chemicals, drugs, which usually operate within the body at a cellular level. Some can be applied externally also and are absorbed through the skin. We will also be concerned with other kinds of intervention which are usually applied externally to affect the nervous system through stimulation of nerve endings. One type of such physical intervention involves invasion, that is surgery.

Following this introduction, there are two parts to the chapter: pharmacology and pain; and physical interventions. In the first section on pharmacology and pain, we shall look at the mechanisms of the various drugs in relation to our understanding of the pain mechanisms. This will prepare the way for the second section where we shall consider the different routes for the administration of drugs; then the different types of drug: mild analgesics; non-steroidal anti-inflammatory drugs (NSAIDs); opiates; and others including combinations and adjuvant drugs. Finally we shall consider the special issues with respect to the use of drugs and infants and children.

In the second part we shall be considering physical interventions, which are generally external applications. These will include transcutaneous electrical nerve stimulation (TENS), counter-irritation, heat and cold, surgery, acupuncture and massage.

THE PHARMACOLOGICAL MANAGEMENT OF PAIN

An important point to make is that the information about the various drugs and treatments is given to illustrate the mechanisms of operation. The information should not be taken as prescriptive of any particular drug or other intervention. Although doses, routes and techniques will be mentioned, the reader is advised to refer to an up-to-date pharmacopoeia or other accurate source of information about drugs and doses. Hospital or other service protocols and guidelines must also be adhered to. Examples given here are for the purposes of illustration only, to show how doses might vary according to route, or different formulation. Similarly the descriptions of physical intervention are brief and should not be seen as the basis for practice. Generally special training is needed before these interventions can be applied. However, it is hoped that sufficient information will be given here to enable an understanding of the process and mechanisms involved, and the circumstances under which particular interventions are most suitable.

How do analgesic drugs work?

There is a wide variety of analgesic drugs available nowadays and all work, basically, by interfering in some way with the transmission of nerve impulses that are interpreted in the brain as pain. The levels in that transmission circuit and the processes involved vary from drug type to drug type. In this section the processes involved in the transmission of the nerve impulse will be rehearsed, with reference back to Chapters 3 and 4, and the way that the various drugs interact with these processes can then be identified.

Peripheral phenomena

Peripheral nerves have their endings in the tissues, the skin, the joints and visceral organs. There they are sensitive to certain changes in their environment which stimulate the electrical nerve impulse which travels along the nerve fibre to its links at synapses with other nerve fibres into the central nervous system. These changes are usually the result of tissue damage caused by external agents or factors, such as heat, chemicals, injury, or by disease.

The tissue damage causes the release of substances that produce the inflammatory response, consisting of redness, swelling, heat and pain. These substances include histamine, bradykinins and what are known as the prostaglandins. The prostaglandins are thought to increase the sensitivity of the nerve endings to bradykinin (McCormack 1994; Wall and Jones 1991) and thus to bring about the nociceptive impulse. Drugs that can interfere with the production of the prostaglandins therefore can have a powerful effect on the transmission of the pain impulse. The C fibres also release chemicals on damage which add to the inflammatory response, for example substance P, neurokinins A and B and other peptides, and the sympathetic nerves release noradrenaline, acetylcholine and adenosine, which also add to the inflammatory process (Melzack and Wall 1996). The synthesis of the prostaglandins seems to be facilitated by the action of cyclo-oxygenase (COX1 and 2) (Yamamoto and Nozaki-Taguchi 1997).

There is one large group of drugs that seems to be able to interfere with the production of the prostaglandins and thus to prevent the generation of the nociceptive impulse. These are the non-steroidal anti-inflammatory drugs (NSAIDs). These drugs play a most important role in the management of pain, particularly with the less severe pain situations, or those associated with inflammation. Their action particularly interferes with the role of the cyclo-oxygenases, and those affecting COX2 seem to be more effective with fewer side effects.

Central phenomena

The signal from the periphery is transmitted further by synapses with neurones in the spinal cord and central nervous system. Synapses are junctions between nerve fibres, whereby the impulse is transmitted from one fibre to the next by the action of chemicals released by the distal fibre and received by the proximal fibre, at special receptor sites (see Figure 3.3). Any other chemical that can be present in the interstitial fluid and inhibit or prevent the reception of the transmitter substance by the proximal fibre will thus interfere with the transmission of the impulse. Nerve cells carry the impulse along by the transfer of sodium and potassium ions across the cell wall. If there is inhibition of this process then no impulse can be transmitted along the nerve fibre.

There are particular sites where such synapses occur, for example in the layers of the dorsal horns of the spinal cord and in the substantia gelatinosa. The reticular formation, the periaqueductal grey and nucleus raphe magnus areas in the midbrain area are also important synaptic sites (Melzack and Wall 1996). The central nervous system itself produces substances that play this role of blocking the transmission, the endorphins, dynorphins and enkephalins, endogenous opiates. These are released by descending fibres and picked up by special receptors on the ascending fibres in the synaptic area.

There are several receptors: mu, delta, kappa, sigma and epsilon (Hughes *et al.* 1975). If the enkephalins are picked up by these receptors, and the mu receptor in particular, the release of the neuro-transmitter substances is inhibited, preventing the onward trans-mission of the signal (McGrath 1990). It was the discovery of the receptors that led to the discovery of the endogenous opiates (Snyder 1980). This action is facilitated by serotonin, a chemical which can also be present in the tissue fluid surrounding the synapse, and which is also released by the descending fibres (Yaksh and Malmberg 1994). It also plays a role in the emotional experience.

Drugs that can similarly be taken up by the opiate receptors or facilitate the action of serotonin can influence the transmission of the nociceptive impulse in the central nervous system. Thus the opiate group of drugs are so influential here that they have given their name to the receptors. The opiates can be administered systemically and have an overall effect or they can be administered regionally at the optimum synaptic area via intrathecal or epidural injection. The drug morphine has a double effect as its breakdown products are also analgesic (British National Formulary 1998). The tricyclic anti-depressants increase the availability of serotonin by inhibiting its re-uptake and so have a direct analgesic action (Botney and Fields 1983). Local anaesthetics inhibit the flow of sodium ions and must be placed in the immediate vicinity of the nerve fibres (Twycross *et al.* 1998).

Routes of administration of analgesics

There are two main types of route for the administration of anal-gesics. The first involves the natural orifices such as the mouth and the anus, utilising the natural permeability of the mucous membranes and gastric and intestinal linings. It also includes the natural perme-ability of the skin. The second involves invasive procedures such as breaking the skin by injections, either into the subcutaneous tissues, the muscles, the veins, or the protective coverings of the spinal cord and central nervous system. It also includes surgery whereby sections of the spinal cord or central nervous system are removed or put permanently or temporarily out of action.

Non-invasive routes

Oral route

This is generally the preferred choice for all drugs. It is particularly recommended for the treatment of cancer pain by the WHO (Hawthorn and Redmond 1998). It is certainly preferred by patients, many of whom find injections painful, particularly children. There can be problems however in the time taken for the drugs to take effect in that the process of absorption from the stomach and gut can be slow (up to an hour). There is also the problem of metabolism of the drug (its breakdown) occurring in the liver before it gets to the tissues where it is needed. Thus not all of the drug gets to the site of the pain and a larger dose may be needed, or the effectiveness is reduced.

Allowing the drug to be absorbed through the buccal or sublingual mucous membranes can enable the drug to get directly into the tissues without the 'first pass' metabolism occurring in the liver.

Rectal route

It can be useful to administer drugs in the form of suppositories if there are problems of gastric side effects. This also avoids the 'first pass' metabolism. However, absorption may be incomplete or erratic (Tempest 1993). NSAIDs particularly can benefit from this route because of potential problems with side effects. However, this route is not so acceptable to patients in the UK, as it is in other countries. It should only be used after careful preparation and parental approval with children.

Transdermal route

Some drugs, if mixed with a suitable cream base, can be absorbed through the skin into the tissues and provide local analgesia. Adhesive patches can also be used, although an initial oral dose may be required to overcome the time lag in absorption. Patches can get over the problem of frequent injections. The cream can be very useful with children or others who do not like injections, as a preparation of the area prior to the injection. However, there is a substantial time lag and good planning is needed.

Invasive routes

Subcutaneous route

Here a needle is inserted into the subcutaneous tissues and the drug is usually administered as a slow continuous infusion. Preferred sites are the subclavicular area, the abdomen, and the anterior chest wall (McCaffrey *et al.* 1994). Single doses are possible of course. Generally the drugs take effect more quickly than the oral route. A wide variety of drugs can be administered in this way. It is very useful if the patient cannot take oral medication.

Intramuscular (IM) route

A much quicker effect is provided by this route. A needle is inserted into one of the large muscles, such as those in the thigh, the vastus lateralis, the buttock-dorsogluteal (although care must be taken not to damage the sciatic nerve). Alternatively the shoulder-deltoid can be used although, as it is a small muscle, only small doses can be given at this site (McCaffrey *et al.* 1994). The injection can itself be painful, and cause local reactions in some people, particularly with NSAIDs (Hawthorn and Redmond 1998).

Intravenous (IV) route

This provides the most rapid effect (almost instantaneously). It is most often used with opioids in emergency situations, or in acute post-operative situations. It can be used for very high doses (McCaffrey *et al.* 1994).

Patient-controlled analgesia

This generally uses the intravenous route and provides a bolus dose when the patient presses a trigger associated with a computer-controlled delivery device. It may be associated with a background infusion, although this is not recommended in the Report of the Royal Colleges (1990). It is mainly used in the post-operative situation, and in some circumstances the subcutaneous route may be used, particularly with patients at home (Heath 1993).

Studies of the relative effectiveness of PCA over other methods of administration vary in their results. For example, in a randomised controlled trial, Berde *et al.* (1993) found that PCA of morphine bolus administration, and PCA of morphine bolus with continuous background low-dose infusion, were both better than IM administration regarding pain relief and satisfaction. Zucker *et al.* (1998) also found a significant difference between PCA and staff-controlled analgesia in a randomised controlled trial following allogenic bone marrow transplantation, regarding pethidine consumption and pain intensity.

However, Snell *et al.* (1997), again in a randomised controlled trial, following abdominal surgery, found no significant differences between PCA and IM with regard to amount of pain, amount of analgesia, satisfaction, time to ambulation and length of stay. They did find that those patients on IM administration required significantly more anti-emetics. Towell (1999) similarly found few differences between PCA and IM from a randomised controlled trial following cardio-thoracic surgery. The assessed variables included: personality (EPQR-A, the revised Eysenck Personality Questionnaire), anxiety (state and trait) pre-operatively; pain at 24 and 48 hrs, anxiety, amount of analgesia, time to extubation, post-operative nausea and vomiting, and length of patient stay, post-operatively. More morphine was administered to/by the PCA group, particularly following transfer to the ward; there was a significant difference in the sensory and affective scores on the Short Form McGill Pain Questionnaire, with the IM group having higher scores. There was greater perception of relief, a shorter time to extubation, less post-operative nausea and vomiting, and a shorter length of patient stay for the PCA group. There was no significant difference between VAS (Visual Analogue Scale) pain scores nor between the anxiety scores. The conclusion was that PCA was a reasonable alternative to IM but it should only be offered as part of a multi-modal range of interventions, depending very much on patient choice.

The conclusion might seem to be that there are many factors operating here and much more research with larger samples over different types of pain are required.

Spinal route (intrathecal)

Here a needle is inserted into the epidural intrathecal or subarachnoid spaces. It is used when side effects from other routes are overwhelming as in cancer sometimes or with post-operative patients (Hawthorn and Redmond 1998). It is recommended for thoracic, orthopaedic and abdominal pain, and leaves the patient more alert, less depressed with less sedative effect and has a longer duration (McCaffrey *et al.* 1994).

Surveys of this route have demonstrated that it can be highly effective. For example, Paice *et al.* (1996) in a survey in the United States found a reduction in pain and an increase in activities of daily living. It was also demonstrated that the reduction in pain was related to an increase in return to work. Winkelmuller and Winkelmuller (1996) similarly found reduction in pain intensity, increase in activity and social relationships, increase in satisfaction and quality of life from a European survey. Reviewing these two studies, Paice *et al.* (1997) argued strongly for the use of intrathecal administration, although they acknowledge problems with catheters and cannulae, as well as with side effects such as constipation, nausea and vomiting, and pruritus.

Intra-articular route

With the knee, particularly following surgery to the joint, such as menisectomy, the intra-articular injection of local anaesthetics and analgesics can be very effective. For example, Rasmussen *et al.* (1998) report a double-blind randomised controlled trial using mixtures of bupivacaine and morphine; bupivacaine, morphine and methylprednisolone; or saline. The bupivacaine and morphine produced reduction in the following: pain on walking and movement, joint effusion, use of crutches and duration of sick leave. With the addition of methylprednisolone there was better relief of pain, less need for additional analgesics, less joint swelling and inflammation, shorter convalescence and increased muscle function. This mixture of nerve block and anti-inflammatory action seems to make an effective combination.

Inhalation

Gases can be absorbed immediately as can very fine sprays of atomised fluids via the respiratory system. NO_2 (nitrous oxide) is being used in cases of heart attack, or injury in accident and emergency departments. It can be used for breakthrough pain in cancer. It is also used in childbirth, in dental surgeries, and for painful investigative procedures. A sufficient dose is given to retain consciousness but to achieve analgesia (Melzack and Wall 1996, citing Sloan 1986 and Fosburg and Crone 1983).

Types of analgesic drugs

As indicated above, this chapter is not offering detailed information about analgesic drugs. It is merely an attempt to illustrate the different types which reflect the modes of action of analgesics. The information has been drawn from sources such as the British National Formulary (1998) and Trounce (1997). The reader is referred to a suitable up-to-date pharmacopoeia, the British National Formulary, hospital and service protocols and guidelines, and the manufacturer's literature.

Mild analgesics

The severity of pain can and does vary from a very mild level to an extreme, unbearable level. Scales as we shall see in Chapter 9 on assessment range from no pain to an upper limit which is usually classified as 'the worst pain I can possibly imagine' or simply 'unbearable'. In many cases the extreme levels of pain are indescribable in words. When we look at mild analgesics we are considering drugs that can be bought 'over the counter' in chemists for self-administration. A popular and effective example is paracetamol.

Paracetamol (acetaminophen) is marketed under a variety of names. It is a particularly useful drug, but does not have a clear mode of action. It seems to be a weak anti-prostaglandin, and to have some central effects which are not fully understood. It has no anti-inflammatory effect like the NSAIDs, and although frequently used as an alternative to aspirin does not work in the same way. Its mode of action seems to be mainly on the central nervous system. It has few side effects, but can have toxic effects on the liver if taken in an overdose, and can cause nausea or a rash. Dosage is usually 500 mg–1g four times in 24 hours in a tablet, capsule, suppository, or elixir formulation. It can be usefully combined with opioids to reduce their dosage as in the analgesic ladder (Kenner 1994; see Figure 7.1). Sometimes classed as an NSAID, paracetamol does not have as strong an anti-inflammatory or anti-prostaglandin action as they do, although it does have an anti-pyretic effect.

Another popular, effective and 'over the counter' analgesic is aspirin (acetylsalicylic acid). It is anti-inflammatory, anti-pyretic as well as analgesic, and acts as an anti-prostaglandin. The popularity of aspirin has taken a knock as a result of its side effects which can be quite severe. These mainly involve its effect on the gastric mucosa causing irritation which can result in bleeding. Some people can have a hypersensitivity reaction. It also has an effect on the blood clotting cascade, and again can cause bleeding through that. It is however used for this anti-coagulant effect in the management of circulatory disorders. These side effects reflect its mode of action and, as always with drugs, there has to be a balance between the benefits from a mode of action and the dangers from the same mode of action.

There are also dangers in using aspirin with children under 12 years of age. It can cause Reye's syndrome which involves brain and liver damage. With adults for whom the gastric and bleeding side effects are not a problem, doses of 300–900 mg four times in 24 hours are recommended, as tablets or rectal suppositories. Overdose can lead to respiratory stimulation, renal failure, pulmonary oedema, convulsions and cardiac arrest.

NSAIDs

Aspirin can be classed with the NSAIDs but tends to be dealt with separately because it is available without prescription, and is such a well-known and popular drug.

There is a wide variety of NSAIDs but they all have generally the same action and effect, in terms of anti-inflammatory, anti-pyretic and analgesic effects. The action and use of the NSAIDs have been extensively reviewed by Moore and McQuay (1988). They play a valuable role in the management of pain and can be more effective than the mild opioids, such as codeine. They tend to operate in the periphery at the site of injury, damage or disease, where an inflammatory response is part of the pain process. Side effects and contra-indications are similar to those for aspirin, but the development of new drugs has led to a reduction in these. The main side effects are gastro-intestinal upset (nausea, diarrhoea), stomach ulcers, bleeding, fluid retention and skin rashes.

MAIN TYPES

The main types include the salicylates (e.g. aspirin); proprionic acid and its derivatives (e.g. ibuprophen); indole acetates (e.g. diclofenac and indomethacine); fenemates (e.g. mefenamic acid); pyrazolones (e.g. azapropazine); and oxicams (e.g. piroxicam). Doses of these drugs are very individual and so are the respective side effects, as different drugs are produced to try to overcome various side effects. For example, aspirin has a recommended dose of 0.3–1 g every four hours, and its side effects have been presented above.

DOSES AND SIDE EFFECTS

Ibuprophen has a recommended dose of 1.2–1.8 mg daily in divided doses, which may be increased to 2.4 mg daily. It has fewer side effects, particularly regarding upper gastro-intestinal side effects, but its anti-inflammatory effects are weaker. Diclofenac with a dose of 75–150 mg daily, and indomethacine with a dose of 50–200 mg daily, have similar action, with indomethacine perhaps being more effective. However, this is at the expense of more side effects, including headaches, dizziness and gastro-intestinal ones. Piroxicam is as effective as diclofenac and has the advantage of a prolonged action, requiring only one dose a day. Its side effects are similar to diclofenac although there may be increased risks of upper gastro-intestinal effects. Mefenamic acid has a dose of 500 mg three times daily. Its side effects include anaemia and thrombocytopaenia, and it can also cause drowsiness, diarrhoea and rashes. Azapropazine has as good an analgesic effect as diclofenac but has a much increased risk of upper gastro-intestinal side effects.

Consultation with up-to-date and individual information about each drug is essential. This is so that the best decision is made about the most suitable drug for any particular patient. Close observation is required regarding side effects so that a change can be made quickly.

Strong analgesics

The opioids

This class of drugs can itself be sub-divided into two levels – mild and strong opioids. They are derivatives of opium, itself derived from the poppy plant, *Papaver somniferum*, or are modern synthetic drugs based on opium. Opium has been in use for thousands of years. Melzack and Wall (1996) report that it was in use in Sumeria 6,000 years ago; that it was used by the Egyptians for sedation more than 3,500 years ago; and that it was prescribed by Galen 1,800 years ago for pain.

In the nineteenth century morphine was isolated as an alkaloid of opium and others followed, such as codeine and papaveretum (Tempest 1993). The discovery of these alkaloids led to attempts to modify them and to the development of drugs with slightly different properties, mainly associated with side effects, duration of effect and route of administration. Examples are heroin, hydromorphine, leverphanol and hydrocodone.

Following further analysis of the structure of morphine and its derivatives, completely artificial drugs have been created in the laboratory, such as meperidine (pethidine), fentanyl, methadone, propoxyphene and pentazocine (Melzack and Wall 1996). Tramadol is another recent development, which seems to have fewer side effects, and its effects are from medium to long duration (British National Formulary 1998). The term opiates is used to describe naturally occurring derivatives of opium, and opioids to describe both naturally occurring and synthetic compounds (Hawthorn and Redmond 1998).

The opioids produce their action by locking onto receptors throughout the body. The majority of receptors have multiple actions, including analgesia, but also other actions which produce the side effects of the drugs. The mu receptors produce respiratory depression, miosis causing blurring of vision, euphoria and consti-pation through inhibition of peristalsis. The kappa receptors produce dysphoria, psychomimetic effects and respiratory depres-sion, whereas the delta receptors produce only analgesia (Hawthorn and Redmond 1998). Other side effects can include suppression of the cough reflex as well as respiratory depression, nausea and vomit-ing, asthma, urticaria, hypotension, difficulty in micturition and/or urinary urgency (Tempest 1993).

Tolerance

Many people, professionals and lay people, have concerns about the use of the opioids in pain management. This is because of fears of respiratory depression, tolerance, dependence and addiction (Levin et al. 1985; Weissman and Dahl 1990). However, respiratory depres-sion is relatively rare. It can easily be treated with naxolone, an opioid antagonist (it replaces the opioid at the receptor sites). Tolerance can occur, as a need for an increasing dose to manage the pain, with the associated fear of not being able to give a large enough dose to achieve the analgesic effect. However, in many instances the pain is increasing as conditions progress and deteriorate, particularly in the longer-term situations. If tolerance does occur then there is rarely any problem in increasing the dose or changing the route of administration. Tolerance to the dangerous side effects such as respiratory depression also occurs and there is no ceiling on the analgesic effects of the opioids (McCaffrey *et al.* 1994).

Dependence and addiction

Three types of dependence have been described – physical, psychological and pharmacological (Tempest 1993). Physical dependence leads to withdrawal symptoms as the body 'misses' the drug. It occurs with drugs other than opioids, such as corticosteroids. It does occur occasionally and the symptoms of withdrawal have been described by Jaffe (1975). They include sweating, runny nose and tears, yawning, nausea and vomiting, diarrhoea, restlessness, tremor, muscle spasm. These can be prevented to a certain extent by phasing the decrease in dose over time. Physical dependence is not addiction.

In psychological dependence there is a need to continue the drug mainly for the psychological effects rather than for any analgesic effect. This is addiction. There is little or no evidence of such dependence occurring in people using opioids for appropriate pain relief. Research indicates that fewer than 1 per cent of patients develop addiction (Marks and Sachar 1973; Jaffe 1975).

McCaffrey *et al.* (1994) write very convincingly of the need to allay misconceptions about pain and its management and in particular about dependence and addiction. They identify and refute several misunderstandings. Prolonged use can be justified because sometimes pain lasts for a long time. Clock watching and/or preferring the needle may mean that there is inadequate relief at the current dosage or route. Seeming to enjoy the drug and to know its name and even dose means that relief is being obtained and we should encourage patients to know about their medication, whatever the type. Requesting the drug in anticipation of pain is no problem as prevention is better than cure, but also the interval may be too long. Finally, requiring higher doses or more frequent doses may mean that tolerance is occurring or that the pain is getting worse.

Pharmacological dependence

This occurs when the body is no longer able to deal with the drugs to achieve the effect and so larger doses are needed (Tempest 1993).

Types of opioid

Mild opioids

The most common mild opioid is codeine (methylmorphine). It is often used as much for its side effects as for its main analgesic effect. For example, it occurs in cough mixtures on account of its anti-tussive effect, and in anti-diarrhoeal medicines because of its constipating effect. It often occurs in cold-relief compound medicines too to cope with headaches and muscle pains. In the body it is converted to norcodeine and morphine which explains its analgesic effect (Findlay *et al.* 1978). A synthetic version is dihydrocodeine, which is not quite so strong and has more side effects (Inturrisi and Hanks 1993). Recommended doses for codeine are 30–60 mg every four hours, and it has relatively few side effects apart from constipation if there is prolonged use. The dose for dihydrocodeine is the same but if the higher doses are used then there tends to be more nausea and vomiting (British National Formulary 1998).

Strong opioids

The main drug in this group is of course morphine. It can be given via all routes and in a variety of formulations including elixirs, immediate and modified release tablets, and suppositories. Oral to parenteral ratio for potency is thought to be 1:3 with chronic pain and 1:6 with acute pain (Tempest 1993; Hanks *et al.* 1996). A usual dose might be 5 mg every three to four hours parenterally. This dose is used as a standard against which the dose of another opioid needed to achieve the same effect is measured – the equianalgesic dose. This is usually provided in the drug literature or in pharmacopoeia.

Doses

A higher dose of some strong opioids is needed to achieve the same effect; others need a lower dose. The dose of fentanyl is 50–200 mg but it is not usually given for long periods. It is used mainly to cover a particular pain episode, such as a procedure. The doses of some morphine derivatives are as follows: heroin (diamorphine), 2.5 mg every three to four hours; hydromorphone 1.3 mg every four hours; papaveretum10–20 mg every three to four hours.

The doses of some synthetic drugs are as follows: pethidine 25–150 mg every three hours; dextropropoxyphene 30–65 mg every three hours; pentazocine (temgesic) 30–60 mg every three to four hours; meptazinol 75–200 mg every three to six hours; and tramadol 50–100 mg every four to six hours. For the longer-acting drugs, for example methadone, the dose is 5–30 mg every six to eight hours; and buprenorphine 0.2–2 mg every six to ten hours. Thus it can be seen that there is a wide variety in the doses required. Therefore it is most important to check a reliable source before giving the drug, and although drug doses may be given in tablets, individual titration must be undertaken for each patient (Twycross and Lack 1990).

Duration of action

The duration of the various opioids vary also. The shortest acting is fentanyl which is perhaps more of a local anaesthetic and only lasts for 10–20 minutes. Most are medium acting, that is for three to four hours on average. In this category are morphine and its derivatives – heroin (diamorphine), papaveretum, hydromorphone, and the synthetic drugs pethidine (meperidine), dextropropoxyphene, pentazocine (fortral).

A very few are long lasting, that is up to six to eight hours, for example methadone, or buprenorphine (Tempest 1993). Following repeated doses there might develop a longer-lasting effect as the breakdown product morphine-6-glucuronide also has an analgesic effect (Hanks *et al.* 1987) which can be increased in patients with renal impairment (Sear *et al.* 1989). The drug tramadol seems to have a duration that lies between the medium and the longer lengths of duration with a dose lasting from four to six hours, as does meptazinol which lasts from three to six hours.

Routes

Most of these drugs can be given by any of the main routes, orally and parenterally. Buprenorphine is broken down in the liver as part of the first pass metabolism (Trounce 1997). Papaveretum is similarly not available in an oral form, and fentanyl can be given by intramuscular injection or by topical application.

Indications

The opioids vary also with regard to the kind of pain. Some are more suitable for the acute situation, for example the peri-operative setting. These include morphine, pethidine, buprenorphine and papaveretum. Fentanyl and morphine can be useful during surgery to improve the level of anaesthesia and reduce the dose of general anaesthetic (British National Formulary 1998). Most of the opioids can be used with moderate to severe pain in the longer term and in palliative care, apart from those mentioned above.

Side effects

Most opioids share the same general side effects, but do vary somewhat in the relative severity of side effects. This is of course the reason why many of them have been developed, to improve the quality of analgesia without also increasing the discomfort to the patient. The main, general side effects of the opioids are nausea and vomiting, constipation and drowsiness. Larger doses can cause respiratory depression and hypotension. Respiratory depression can usually be reversed by the administration of naxalone, an antagonist.

Other side effects include difficulty with micturition, biliary and ureteric spasm, sympathetic reactions such as dry mouth, sweating, tachycardia and palpitations. There may also be miosis, bradycardia, hypotension, or hypothermia. Rashes, urticaria or pruritus may occur. Effects on the central nervous system may include hallucinations, dysphoria, mood changes, or decreased libido. In the longer term there may develop dependence.

The individual drugs can vary regarding the number and/or degree of side effects. Morphine for example also can cause a state of euphoria and mental detachment. Buprenorphine has abuse potential, can cause severe vomiting, and its effects are only partially reversed by naxalone. Codeine has severe constipating effects as noted above and thus is not suitable for longer-term use. Dihydrocodeine has similar analgesic effects to codeine, but can have more serious side effects such as nausea and vomiting. Dextropropoxyphene is often combined with paracetamol but as such can cause serious effects if overdosed. These are respiratory depression, heart failure and hepatotoxicity.

Diamorphine (heroin) can cause less nausea and hypotension than morphine. Pethidine is less constipating than morphine, and meptazinol has a low incidence of respiratory depression, but it does cause nausea and vomiting. Methadone is less sedating than morphine. The relatively new drug tramadol has less respiratory depression, less constipation and less addiction potential, but can cause psychiatric reactions. Pentazocine also can cause hallucinations and thought disturbances, and is not recommended if there is a history of myocardial infarction.

Combinations of drugs and adjuvant drugs

Some of the milder analgesic drugs can be given in combination to try to achieve a stronger effect. They usually comprise a weak opioid and aspirin or paracetamol. Some are available 'over the counter'. Examples are co-codamol (codeine and paracetamol); co-codaprin (codeine and aspirin); co-dydramol (dihydrocodeine and paracetamol); co-proxamol (dextropropoxyphene and paracetamol); codafen (ibuprofen and codeine). The British National Formulary lists some hundreds of preparations of 'over the counter' combinations containing aspirin, paracetamol, and/or others such as codeine, caffeine and ephedrine type drugs to alleviate the symptoms of colds such as a runny nose. It is important to ensure that those prescribing drugs or administering them are aware of the possible effects of self-administered drugs such as these on top of the prescribed drugs.

Moore et al. (1997) have reviewed randomised controlled trials of paracetamol alone and in combination with codeine for acute pain. They identified a total of 63 trials some of which also included placebo. They found that overall the addition of codeine to paracetamol led to 12 per cent more patients gaining more than 50 per cent pain relief. They argue that although paracetamol is itself a strong and useful analgesic the addition of 60 mg codeine seems to be worthwhile. However, these combinations, particularly those with codeine and paracetamol, can have very serious overdose effects. Respiratory depression can be fatal particularly if the drug is taken with alcohol (Tempest 1993). There may also be allergic reactions, and the addition of the opioid codeine brings the full range of opioid side effects with it, particularly constipation. The elderly are particularly vulnerable (British National Formulary 1998).

Mixtures known as 'cocktails', such as the 'Brompton Cocktail', are frequently made up for patients in severe pain and in a terminal situation (Melzack et al. 1976). These contain such drugs as morphine, cocaine, with gin and honey. This gives a narcotic and stimulant effect. They may also contain phenothiazines. Rasmussen *et al.* (1998) have developed a mixture of hormone (glucocorticoid) and analgesic (bupivacaine and morphine) which reduces the inflammatory response, pain and convalescence after arthroscopic menisectomy.

The analgesic ladder

The World Health Organisation (WHO 1996) has argued for the use of what is known as the analgesic ladder, particularly when dealing with increasing or very severe pain. By this is meant a stepped approach to the use of analgesics, starting with the milder types and then adding to them the stronger ones. Thus one would start with paracetamol adding NSAIDs to increase the effect. If these were not enough then one could add the mild opioids proceeding to the strong opioids as necessary. If the patient was immediately or already in very severe pain then one would go straight to a strong drug. However, with a moderate to severe pain, one would start with the milder drugs, assessing the response from the patient, using some quantitative measurement of the pain and step up the ladder until a satisfactory level of pain control had been achieved (see Figure 7.1). Mainly derived for the management of cancer pain, it is also recommended wherever long-term and varying degrees of pain might be experienced (Hawthorn and Redmond 1998).

This ladder demonstrates a different form of drug combination to that described above, whereby different kinds of drugs are given together to enhance the analgesic effect. As has been emphasised above it is vitally important that each individual patient being treated for pain in this way must have a careful titration of these increasing combinations, involving careful and regular recorded assessment of their effect on the patient's pain. It is often a question of professional experience which suggests the particular combination of drugs to offer the patient.

Adjuvant drugs

There are quite a few drugs, developed for other purposes, that have been found to enhance the analgesic effect. These are now known as adjuvant drugs and are administered with the traditional analgesics to give an enhanced effect. As indicated above they may be added to the analgesic ladder. Drugs from a variety of groups, such as

Step 1 Mild pain	Step 2 Moderate pain	Step 3 Severe pain
Non-opioids	*Non-opioids*	*Non-opioids*
• paracetamol • NSAIDs	• paracetamol • NSAIDs	• paracetamol • NSAIDs
	Mild opioids	*Mild opioids*

	• codeine and/or
	  diclofenac
		• codeine and/or
		  diclofenac

		Strong opioids

		• morphine
		  • epidural infusion
		  • subcutaneous
		    infusion
		  • IV injection
		  • NCA
		  • PCA

Adjuvant drugs could be given as well at each step

Figure 7.1   The analgesic ladder

anti-depressants, anti-convulsants, neuroleptics, muscle relaxants and anti-emetics, are used. Some do seem to have an independent analgesic effect, such as the tricyclic anti-depressants. Where the drugs are used to relieve pain they are sometimes known as co-analgesics. If they are mainly used to deal with side effects or other symptoms, thus helping in the overall management of the pain situation, then they are known as adjuvant medications (McCaffrey *et al.* 1994). Situations where there is depression, anxiety or difficulty in sleeping may call for the use of adjuvant medication.

The use of these drugs, as well as the use of combinations of analgesics, allows a very individual approach to the management of pain. More aspects of the pain experience can be tackled with this wider range of pharmacological preparations.

Anti-depressants

The tricyclic group of anti-depressants do seem to have a separate analgesic effect, which has been known of for some time, as demonstrated in a review by Monks and Merskey (1984), and also by Stauffer (1987), among others. An example is amitriptyline at a dose of 10–25 mg up to 150 mg. Its side effects include drowsiness and dry mouth with blurred vision, palpitations and dizziness. It is frequently given at night when the drowsiness can be useful and the other side effects are not so disruptive. It is mainly used with neuropathic pain, such as trigeminal neuralgia or diabetic neuropathy (British National Formulary 1998). The dose to achieve analgesia is usually lower than that to achieve an anti-depressant effect. It is thought to work by stimulating the release of endogenous analgesics through increasing the amount of serotonin and similar amines in the central nervous system and also by preventing their breakdown (McCaffrey *et al.* 1994; Melzack and Wall 1996). These anti-depressants may also be called upon to treat depression if it occurs along with the pain, particularly with chronic pain.

Another group of drugs which can be helpful with similar neuropathic pain is the anti-convulsants (Swerdlow 1984). An example is carbamazepine, with a dose of 100 mg once or twice a day up to 200 mg taken three to four times daily. This effect is thought to be achieved by reduction of neuronal excitability.

The neuroleptic group of drugs is helpful when there is an associated anxiety state, or an anti-emetic is required. They can also have a muscle relaxant action. They are thought to be more effective when given with anti-depressants or opioids (Hawthorn and Redmond 1998). Examples are chlorpromazine with a dose of 10–25 mg every four to six hours; haloperidol, 0.5–2 mg as an anti-emetic. The benzodiazepines are occasionally used, such as diazepam, but there are great dangers of addiction with this group and there may be depression and an increase in the pain (Melzack and Wall 1996), and great care is recommended (Tempest 1993).

Occasionally a muscle-relaxant effect is required where muscular tension or spasm is part of the pain phenomenon. An example is the drug baclofen, at a dose of 5 mg three times a day. Diazepam again is useful here, and has been shown to have an analgesic effect (Hawthorn and Redmond 1998), although the warning of Tempest (1993) still applies. Smooth muscle relaxants have a place too, and examples are hyoscine at 20 mg, four times a day; alverine at 60–120 mg one to three times daily; and mebeverine 135 mg one to three times a day. They are particularly useful for pain in the gastro-intestinal tract. They have side effects of blurred vision and dry mouth (British National Formulary 1998).

Corticosteroids have been shown to be effective with regard to cancer pain. They also reduce oedema and thus can contribute to pain relief. Dexamethasone is a popular choice with a dose of 0.4–4 mg by intra-articular injection for joint pain, or 0.5–10 mg daily orally. These drugs have many side effects, including on the gastro-intestinal tract, the musculo-skeletal system, the endocrine system, neuropsychiatric effects and ophthalmic effects. It is recommended that the minimum dose is given for the shortest possible time to achieve the desired effect (British National Formulary 1998).

Pharmacology and pain in children

Evidence is quoted in the introduction that there is still a tendency to under-prescribe and administer analgesics, or even not to prescribe or administer analgesics to young children and infants (see also Goldschneider (1998) who argues that there is evidence that this can have long-term effects on the individual). Nevertheless, the same kinds of drugs used with adults can be used, generally, with children and infants. However, there are some limitations and problems associated with medication of the young and these are to be considered in this section. There is still evidence that frequently PRN prescriptions lead to under-administration by nurses (Hamers *et al.* 1998). The authors, following a review, recommend that a specific standard prescription is given rather than PRN. This point will be referred to again in Chapter 10 when we consider aspects of the administration of treatments.

An argument is made for keeping the pharmacological management of pain in children simple by limiting the drugs used to a well-proven few (Twycross *et al.* 1998). They suggest paracetamol, diclofenac, codeine phosphate and morphine. They also suggest a simple but effective analgesic ladder suitable for children, but following the same principles of that for adults (WHO 1990). McCaffrey *et al.* (1994) recommend a pharmacopoeia for children, such as the *Paediatric Vade Mecum* (1993).

Routes

Generally the same routes can be used for children as for adults. The oral route is to be preferred as most children hate injections. However, this route is not effective if the child is vomiting. There is also a time lag and there may be fluctuations in level (Twycross *et al.* 1998). Suppositories are also not liked and care must be taken in seeking permission from parents. Subcutaneous and intravenous infusions are more acceptable once the needle/cannula is in place and PCA is possible from the age of 7 years, and even earlier use has been reported (see Carter (1994) for a review). The topical application EMLA cream (eutetic mixture of local anaesthetics) is a useful way of easing procedures (Halperin *et al.* 1989), although pre-planning is essential as it takes 60–90 minutes to take effect. It is not recommended for neonates unfortunately as it does not reduce the trauma. Other topical applications are available such as lignocaine cream and spray. These are much faster in their action but of shorter duration also. They are useful for such procedures as urethral catheterisation (Twycross *et al.* 1998).

Types of analgesic

Mild analgesics

The NSAIDs and paracetamol are useful with children and a variety of formulations are available, particularly for oral or rectal adminis-tration. Paracetamol can be given at various doses depending on the age of the infant or child. McCaffrey *et al.* (1994) recommend the following: 2–3 mths, 60 mg in a single dose a day; 3–12 mths, 60–125 mg; 1–5 yrs, 125–250 mg; 6–12 yrs, 250–500 mg; above 12 yrs, 500–1,000 mg.

Aspirin (acetylsalicylic acid) is not given to children under the age of 12 yrs, as Reye's syndrome may develop (rarely), which involves the brain and the liver and is fatal. There are also the dangers of bleeding as indicated with adult administration.

The NSAIDs such as diclofenac are very popular for chronic pain, although there is little evidence of their efficacy with acute pain (Carter 1994). It has fewer side effects than aspirin. A dose of 1 mg/kg every eight hours is recommended.

Strong analgesics

The opioids

There is little research studying the administration of the opioids to children, nevertheless there is much empirical evidence to confirm the general safety of these drugs, if monitored carefully. Dahlstrom *et al.* (1979) demonstrate that children metabolise opioids in the same way that adults do, and that they are no more sensitive to them than adults. Kaiko (1980) found that the half life of opioids varies with the age of the child and the dosage. Nevertheless it was argued as long ago as 1983 by Miser *et al.* that they can be given by continuous infusion or syringe pump to children with terminal cancer. However, Llewellyn (1997) argues that in infants and neonates there is reduced clearance of morphine and thus a tendency for the level of the drug to build up in the body and to take longer for the level to come down on cessation of the infusion (Goldman and Lloyd-Thomas 1991). De Veber (1986) reports that some children with chronic cancer pain may need a higher dose.

Synthetic opioids such as methadone seem to have advantages offering fewer side effects and longer duration than morphine (Berde *et al.* 1988). Cocktails of drug mixtures, as described above for adults, are also available for children. However, some children may reject them if they contain alcohol (Twycross 1979). Mixtures more attractive to children can be made up (P. A. McGrath 1990).

Mild opioids – codeine

Codeine is up to 1/6th weaker than morphine and therefore is less prone to side effects such as respiratory depression or constipation (Twycross *et al.* 1998). A recommended dose is 1 mg/kg every four hours. It may be found in combination with other drugs such as paracetamol.

Strong opioids – morphine

There is no difference in sensitivity to morphine between children of different ages (Dahlstrom *et al.* 1979), although Twycross *et al.* (1998) claim that neonates are more sensitive, drawing particularly on the work of Morselli *et al.* (1980). They argue that this is because they have a higher proportion of endogenous opioids; a reduced blood brain barrier which means that more gets through; a greater variation in receptor type; reduced ability to bind morphine to plasma proteins and therefore there is a larger amount free; and similarly there is a reduced ability to metabolise morphine and therefore it stays in the body longer. Doses for children over 6 months increase from 0.1 mg/kg to 0.2 mg/kg at 12 yrs every four hours (orally or parenterally). Twycross *et al.* (1998) recommend that for neonates a dose of 0.01 mg/kg/hr should be used with very careful monitoring. In spite of the evidence that neonates are perhaps more vulnerable to the effects of morphine, Carter (1994) also argues that this is no reason for hesitancy in using an appropriate dose for neonatal pain, with careful observation. This author also offers a very thorough review of the management of pain in neonates.

The same side effects operate with infants and children as with adults. Nausea and vomiting, constipation and respiratory depression are the main ones. The nausea and vomiting frequently interfere with oral administration.

Fentanyl, a synthetic opioid, is frequently used with children. It has a rapid onset. When given intravenously its effects can be experienced after as little as two to three minutes. It is of short duration and therefore is good for procedural pain, and in accident and emergency situations. It is much more potent than morphine (Roop Moyer and Howe 1991) and is available in lollipop formulation for oral and transmucosal use (Schechter *et al.* 1990).

Herbal medicine

The use of plants or extracts from plants for medicinal purposes has been known since Neanderthal times. The use of herbal medicines for the treatment of pain has had a high priority during this time and many herbs are now known which have analgesic actions (Lewith *et al.* (1996) have reviewed this and a variety of other complementary therapies). There is a Chinese and a western version of knowledge about the use of herbs in medicine. The philosophy behind both is to promote the individual's own self-healing ability. In the western version the medicines are derived entirely from plant material, whereas the Chinese medicines also incorporate animal and mineral materials. Examples of some herbal medicines related to the management of pain include feverfew (*Tanacetum partenium*) for migraine; St John's Wort (*Hypericum perforatum*) which has an anti-inflammatory action, as well as mild sedative and analgesic actions; Valerian root which has sedative and tranquillising properties; and ginger, which is well known for its anti-emetic action (Lewith *et al.* 1996).

Conclusion

The pharmacology of pain management has a long history and the story is continuing to develop as more and more research and development goes into new drugs and formulations. However, the main types of drug are well established and, generally, very effective. The drugs work in different ways but always relate to the underlying mechanisms and process of the pain experience as described in previous chapters. The range of strengths, types and mechanisms utilised by the drugs should ensure that for most people in pain there is a feasible pharmacological strategy of care. This variety also makes it possible for a very individualised programme of care to be devised for patients. It also enables this strategy to be changed as the person's condition or pain experience changes.

However, there are also other methods of approaching pain, those utilising physical procedures and processes which can add to the effectiveness of a pain-management programme. These will be presented in the second section of this chapter.

PHYSICAL INTERVENTIONS FOR PAIN

There has been a long history of attempts to relieve or to ease pain by using non-pharmacological methods. In this section we shall be reviewing some of the main ones that do seem to have some evidence to support their continued use. Some are very old methods such as massage and aromatherapy, the application of heat and cold, or acupuncture; and others are relatively new such as surgery and the permanent or temporary inactivation of nerves, and the application of a mild electrical current to the skin.

How do the physical methods work?

With surgery and the inactivation of nerves there is the obvious physical disruption of the flow of impulses to the central nervous system and the awareness of pain. The destruction of peripheral nerves can be achieved by the application of phenol, alcohol or freezing, or by surgically severing them (Melzack and Wall 1996). There do seem to be problems with these approaches in that all too frequently the pain recurs and not infrequently it is more severe. This seems to be the result of other pathways developing to carry the impulses, or by links developing with nerves supplying another area. The full explanation however is still not available (Melzack and Wall 1996).

The other physical methods seem to largely operate by bringing about the stimulation of the large diameter fibres which then have the effect of closing the gate and preventing the transmission of the pain impulses up the ascending system to the higher centres. There is a possibility that they also cause the release of endorphins. Some may act as a counter-irritant, or distraction, and others, such as heat, by facilitating muscle relaxation, and blood flow which can facilitate healing locally. There is an increase in the local circulation of blood which causes reddening and an increase in the removal of waste products (Horrigan 1993). Cold can also act by reducing swelling through causing vasoconstriction and thus reducing the release of fluids into the tissues, and the inflammatory response. It can also cause numbness if cold enough, which prevents the flow of electrical impulses along the nerve fibres (Horrigan 1993).

Acupuncture is thought to work by stimulating certain points on the surface of the body, under the skin, through needles which link with channels of energy flow called meridians. It has been a mainstay of Chinese medicine for thousands of years. The action of twirling or otherwise stimulating the needles is thought to effect a redressing of the balance between opposing aspects of the energy forces, the Yin and the Yang. In terms of western medicine there seems to be a possibility that the action stimulates the release of endorphins or inhibits the flow of pain impulses through closing the gate (Mayer *et al.* 1976). This is supported by the fact that it seems to be the stimulation that causes the effect rather than the particular site (Lewit 1979). The effect also seems to be related to the intensity of the stimulation and its effect on the descending inhibitory system, involving the periaqueductal grey matter (Soper and Melzack 1982; Le Bars *et al.* 1983; and see Melzack and Wall 1996). Knardahl *et al.* (1998) have shown that electro-acupuncture can increase the pain threshold paralleled by a significant increase in muscular sympathetic nerve activity.

Types of physical treatment

Permanent or temporary inactivation of nerves

This can be carried out by surgical or chemical means. With surgery the actual nerve fibres are cut, or sections are excised. It can involve the ascending peripheral nerves, the nerve roots, the sympathetic nervous system (sympathectomy), or the spinal cord itself (cordotomy). The problem with the peripheral nerves is that they also contain the motor fibres and so there will also tend to be a paralysis of the affected area. An operation known as rhizotomy involves separating the motor and sensory fibres at the root before they enter the single peripheral nerve structure. This is a much more delicate procedure. It is perhaps most useful when there is an obvious physical cause, such as compression of a nerve, or distension of an organ (Hawthorn and Redmond 1998).

With a cordotomy the ventro-lateral ascending spino-thalamic tract is severed. As indicated above however there is frequently a recurrence of the pain. This is thought to occur through a variety of mechanisms. These include the generation of nervous sprouts at the severed end which are hypersensitive. Synapses may develop with other nerve endings via these sprouts. There seem to be chemical changes in the nerve itself, and it seems also to become more sensitive to chemicals from the sympathetic nerves. The cessation of impulses from the severed nerve may release or reveal previously inhibited signals from another source (see Melzack and Wall 1996). However, if the treatment is carried out with a needle and heat via a wire down the needle to gain very accurate placing of the oblation, then a more effective outcome can be achieved (Ischia et al. 1985). This approach is perhaps best in terminal care when the recurrence of pain may come too late.

As well as cutting the nerve fibres they may be inactivated by chemicals, such as phenol or alcohol, or more temporarily by the application of local anaesthetic or an analgesic. Nevertheless with these permanent forms of treatment there remains this problem of an eventual return of even more severe pain. The use of local anaesthetics and even analgesics to provide temporary nerve block is an increasing development in the management of pain and in the performance of various procedures, even surgery (Cousins and Bridenbaugh 1987). These have been discussed under the pharmacological heading in this chapter.

Cutaneous stimulation – massage

This term includes such activities as touching and stroking as well as the formal process of massage. It involves the stimulation of the skin and underlying tissues to provide comfort and relief from pain (see review by Haldeman 1994). It usually involves stroking and the application of varying degrees of pressure to the skin. It causes feelings of warmth and comfort (Doehring 1989), muscular relaxation, distraction, interpersonal communication through touch and improves the circulation (Mobily *et al.* 1994). It can involve only part of the body, such as the hand, the face and neck, the back or larger areas. There is little experimental research to confirm its use. It has such a long history and is practised so widely with obvious positive effect that it seems almost unnecessary. However, some anecdotal descriptions of its effects have been published such as Sims (1986); Ferrel-Torry and Glick (1993) with cancer patients; and Davies and Riches (1995) with rheumatoid arthritis (see Hawthorn and Redmond 1998).

Vibration may also be applied as cutaneous stimulation. This may be hand-held or with pads. McCaffrey *et al.* (1994) recommend it for muscle pain, tension headache, rheumatoid arthritis, for example, as well as neuropathic pain and phantom limb pain. They recommend electric vibrators, some of which can be strapped to the hand which is then held over the body part. They cite Lundeberg (1984) and Shere *et al.* (1986) as demonstrating pain relief. Training is usually recommended before one attempts to undertake massage for pain relief.

Patients receiving therapeutic touch, involving a non-touch technique, have been shown to have significantly reduced pain ratings and a reduction in anxiety compared with a sham therapeutic touch group, in a randomised controlled trial (Turner *et al.* 1998). The therapeutic touch technique involves holding the hands two to five inches above the patient's skin and thus 'the practitioner consciously directs or sensitively modulates the person's energies' (p. 12).

Aromatherapy

This is a form of treatment using essential oils extracted from plants for therapeutic effect (Stevenson 1995). It is often used with massage which usually involves some oil, talcum powder, or soapy water, as a lubricant to facilitate the movement of the hands over the skin. A base oil can have added to it a more aromatic oil so that the perfume can also create an effect. Such aromatic oils can also be vaporised, heated, or added to a warm bath to create their effect. Aromatic oils such as rose, lavender, jasmine have a relaxing effect;

black pepper, rosemary, juniper have a more warming effect. Lavender can also be used for first-aid for burns and for relieving discomfort after childbirth. Neroli is often used for anxiety.

There is little evidence to support the use of aromatic oils in this way. Nevertheless anecdotal reports indicate that they can be soothing and comforting. The patient should always be the one to determine whether the effect is pleasant or comforting (Stevensen 1995). For aching joints a warm bath with rosemary, bergamot or camomile is recommended; for dysmenorrhoea or constipation, warm compresses and gentle massage with camomile or lavender. Cold compresses with lavender or peppermint are recommended for headache and with lavender or camomile for sprains (Horrigan 1993). It is important that the necessary training for this treatment should be undertaken prior to using it.

Heat

Heat has been used with warm baths, both artificial and naturally occurring, over the centuries. There are many ways in which heat can be applied. Hot water bottles, packs, dry and wet compresses can be applied locally. Radiant heat can be applied over an area using a light bulb; immersion, total or partial, in a warm bath can be used. Many of these applications are suitable for use in the home. They can be very helpful with muscle spasm, joint stiffness, low back pain, menstrual cramps. They also facilitate relaxation (Mobily *et al.* 1994). Heat improves the blood flow as indicated above, but care must be taken where there is danger of causing further damage, such as where there is swelling, impaired sensation, drowsiness, poor blood supply and superficial malignancy (McCaffrey *et al.* 1994).

Deep heat can be applied using ultrasound, diathermy (microwaves or short-wave radio), or infra-red radiation. This can be very helpful with deep-seated pain, and joints. However, this sort of treatment is usually provided by professionals with special training, such as physiotherapists.

Cold

The application of cold, as packs or compresses, has been shown to cause vasoconstriction, and reduce swelling and the amount of metabolites in the tissues (Ernst and Fialka 1994), as in sprains, bursitis and myofibrositis (McCaffrey *et al.* 1994). It also helps in the reduction of muscle spasm, muscle tone, spasticity and joint stiffness (Ross and Soltes 1995). Cold may be applied through icepacks, ethylchloride spray, immersion in cold water with ice, or by the application of a pack of frozen food such as frozen peas. A compress made with lightly wrung out towel and cold water can be effective. It can be helpful to grease the skin so that it does not get soggy (Horrigan 1993). Generally one should not use direct ice or freezing or near freezing temperatures. However, Melzack and Wall argue for the therapeutic use of ice as a form of hyperstimulation analgesia. The production of pain from the deep cold of the ice at certain trigger points has been shown to provide relief from acute pain (Melzack *et al.* 1980).

Transcutaneous electrical nerve stimulation

A process of cutaneous stimulation that seems to be very effective and is now well established is that of transcutaneous electrical nerve stimulation (TENS). Developed by Wall and Sweet from the basic principles of the Gate Control Theory (1967) it involves the electrical stimulation of the large low threshold fibres through the skin. According to the theory (Melzack and Wall 1965), the stimulation of the large low threshold fibres should result in action in the dorsal horn where there is inhibition of afferent pain impulses (see Chapter 3). The electrical current is supplied by a battery-powered impulse generator. This transmits the impulses via wires or leads to the electrodes that are placed over the painful area. The electrodes usually consist of squares of flexible conducting silicone, two to three inches square. Using conducting jelly they are stuck to the skin with adhesive tape or they may be self-adhesive (see Figure 7.2). The impulse consists of low-voltage current applied for 40–500 microseconds at a rate of 2–250 Hz (per second), a common rate being 100–500 microsecond pulses at 40–70 Hz (see Woolf and Thompson (1994) for a review).

The patient experiences a tingling or vibrating sensation and is recommended to experiment with the placing of the electrodes to obtain the maximum effect. The strength, pattern, period and rate of the impulses can be adjusted to generate the best result. This is very much a patient-controlled method of pain relief. There is much evidence now to show that this method is effective for a variety of chronic pain situations. These include neurogenic pain (Bates and

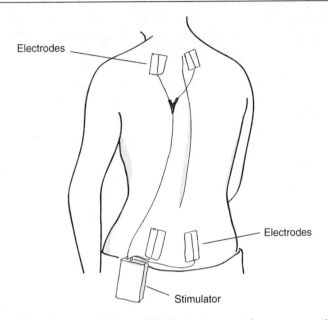

Figure 7.2   Diagram showing a TENS stimulator, with some examples of electrode positioning

Mathan 1980) and chronic back pain (Eriksson *et al.* 1979). Many patients obtain total or major pain relief which can outlast the period of stimulation (Johnson *et al.* 1991). It has been used with acute pain for such situations as trauma. Sprains, torn muscles, fractured ribs and even acute arthritic pain have been successfully treated in this way (Woolf and Thompson 1994), as well as post-operative pain.

When used for a long period it does seem that tolerance can occur (Bates and Mathan 1980; Johnson *et al.* 1991). This may be the result, as with pharmacological preparations, of a worsening of the pain. However, some patients do seem to develop tolerance. Attempts to change the frequency and/or rate can help, but another form of analgesia may be necessary. Care must be taken with patients with pacemakers, or other cardiac problems or in pregnancy, although for labour pain it can be very useful (Woolf and Thompson 1994). It should not be used on the neck, particularly the anterior part, because it might cause hypotension as a result of an effect on the vagal nerve.

Acupuncture

Reaching Europe in the second half of the seventeenth century from the Far East by workers for the Dutch East India Company, acupuncture has been practised widely since then (Campbell 1987). Although originating in Chinese medicine, there have been many attempts to correlate it with western medicine. This applies particularly to the experience of pain. The discovery of the endorphins and enkaphalins have helped to provide a rationale for the effects gained with the management or prevention of pain through the use of acupuncture (Mayer *et al.* 1976; Melzack and Wall 1996).

Needles are inserted into what are known as trigger points, and they are rotated gently or have low voltage electrical stimulation applied to them. Pressure on these trigger points has also been shown to have an effect. Melzack *et al.* (1977) identified trigger points with acupuncture points. In reviews of the effects of acupuncture on pain (Melzack 1994; Melzack and Wall 1996) there is clear evidence of its effectiveness against pain. Evidence seems to confirm that it is the act of stimulation that creates the effect rather than the particular site (Frost *et al.* 1980). It is thought that the effect is generated by activating the brain stem and thus stimulating the descending diffuse noxious inhibitory controls. These also involve the periaqueductal grey matter, which seems to have a somatotopic organisation (Soper and Melzack 1982).

Physical treatments and children

All of the above treatments are suitable for use with children (Carter 1994; Twycross *et al.* 1998). The child should be old enough to understand the instructions or what is being done, perhaps with the help of parents. Indeed some of the interventions can usefully employ parents in helping in the care of their child. Even TENS has been used effectively. However, there is little experimentally controlled research, although anecdotal evidence suggests that it can bring relief (Eland 1993). The child can be involved here as this is very much a patient-controlled process. Parents again can help the child.

With massage care must be taken to obtain permission of the child and parent, and the child can be involved with decision making about the site and kind of massage to be used (Carter 1994). It may also be used with aromatic oils, for example lavender (Davis 1988b). McGrath *et al.* (1993) argue against the use of excessive touch and physical stimulation with neonates as this can cause stress rather than relieve it (Wolke 1987).

The use of nerve blocks and topical anaesthesia has been recommended for children (P. A. McGrath 1990), and the latter can play an important role in the prevention of procedural pain.

Conclusion

A variety of methods have been identified as offering alternative or adjunctive support for the management of pain. There seem to be good scientific rationales for each of them, utilising Gate Control Theory and the existence of endogenous inhibitory and analgesic processes and substances. Many of these interventions can be patient controlled or involve parents, spouses or friends. They certainly offer nursing and other health-care professionals a wider range of interventions than just the usual pharmacological ones. These physical interventions are usually applied alongside or in support of the latter. Most of them require little specialist equipment, apart from TENS or the use of aromatic oils. Most however do require specialist training in their use. All should be considered as possibilities in providing a balanced plan of care in both the acute and chronic pain situations. The use of what are called the complementary therapies is somewhat debatable although many people in pain do gain relief of some sort or other from their use. Herbert (1998) has argued very strongly for their use in accident and emergency settings where the administration of analgesics may not be advocated or there may be long periods of waiting for assessment.

Chapter 8

Psychological interventions

> The labour we delight in physics pain.
>
> Shakespeare

Introduction

In our analysis of the pain experience we have identified various aspects: the sensory-discriminative, the motivational-emotional, the psychological, and the social-cultural. In this chapter we shall be looking at interventions that relate to the psychological and social mechanisms of the pain experience. Some aspects have already been touched on in the discussion of pharmacological and physical interventions which themselves have an effect on the emotional aspects. In particular this relates to the emotional aspects such as anxiety and motivation by helping the person in pain to cope more effectively with the pain. By reducing anxiety and increasing coping ability, motivation to continue with treatment can be maintained.

There are three main approaches to the psychological management of pain. The first is to bring about psycho-physiological changes for primarily an emotional effect although there may also be a physiological analgesic effect. This involves mainly various strategies to bring about relaxation. The second is to distract the mind from the pain experience, which may facilitate the first; and the third is to change the meaning of the pain. This latter involves two separate aspects. The first is the reinterpretation of the pain and by thinking more positively about it facilitate coping or motivation. The second is to learn more positive adaptive behaviours in response to the pain experience. We shall be looking at each of these approaches in turn in the following sections of this chapter. First however we shall look at how it is thought that the various treatments work.

How do psychological interventions work?

Relaxation has a powerful effect generally on various systems in the body and pain relief is one of these. By encouraging and facilitating muscular and mental relaxation there are definite effects created by changes in the sympathetic nervous system which have a direct action on the pain mechanisms (Benson *et al.* 1984). Tension itself can increase pain, particularly such as tension headaches, and pain associated with joints and muscles (Jessup and Gallegos 1994). The relaxation also has an effect on anxiety. By reducing anxiety, which utilises the same parts of the midbrain as the ascending and descending pain mechanisms such as the limbic system, the thalamus, and the reticular formation, there is a direct physiological link to these pain mechanisms (Melzack and Wall 1996).

Distraction seems to raise the perception threshold and prevent the acknowledgement of pain impulses (Fellner 1971), and thus increase the tolerance of pain (Scott and Barber 1977). Thus it is more of a coping strategy. Similarly the reinterpretation of the pain experience can help people to cope with it more effectively. Thinking of the pain in a more positive light or a less threatening light can facilitate motivation to change lifestyle or to continue other pain-management strategies (Edgar 1993). There can also be a direct link with the emotions, anxiety and depression (Fishman and Loscalzo 1987; Ciccone and Grzesiak 1988), and through a reduction of anxiety help both to cope and bring about pain reduction.

It is argued that much of people's pain behaviour is negative and is learned throughout life (Fordyce 1976). By unlearning these maladaptive behaviours and learning new adaptive, positive behaviours, the person in pain can experience more positive feelings about the pain and develop a more constructive approach to his or her pain and lifestyle. This approach is based on the theory of operant conditioning. According to this, behaviour is repeated and learned through the effect of reinforcers. A reinforcer is anything that increases the likelihood of the behaviour being repeated and so learned. A variety of types of reinforcement for pain behaviour has been identified (Turk and Flor 1987). The theory of operant conditioning is based on the early work of Skinner (e.g. 1938, 1953), and the involvement of the emotions seems to be crucial in humans (Dollard and Miller 1950; Wachtel 1977; Gray 1990).

Relaxation

Relaxation has already been mentioned as the possible outcome of some of the physical treatments discussed in the previous chapter. The techniques used in this chapter do not depend on the application of any physical intervention, but can produce physical relaxation. By relaxation is meant freedom from mental or physical stress or tension. It is an active process demanding concentration. The main approach involves achieving physical relaxation by asking the patient to gradually relax all skeletal muscles often from the toes upwards. This system was first introduced for the management of pain by Jacobson in 1938. His approach was for the patient to relax one muscle at a time. This was very time consuming although effective. However, modifications to the method include the use of groups of muscles together to speed up the process (Benson 1975; Benson *et al.* 1977). The process may involve tensing the muscles first prior to relaxing them. However, care must be taken here if the pain is associated with tension or joints as tensing the muscle might in fact increase the pain. This approach is based on meditative practices and involves also breathing exercises and focused attention.

Imagery and relaxation

The procedure can also be of a more psychological nature, by relying on the patient's ability, perhaps with training to use his or her imagination to aid relaxation. Thus by imagining scenes, sounds, or experiences that can distract from the pain situation and have as a major component a sense of relaxation and positive well-being, the process of physical relaxation can be facilitated.

Although the process demands concentration and participation it is essentially an attempt to achieve passivity. It cannot be forced. The therapist usually gives instructions in a quiet calm way, and in a relaxing, quiet setting. However, the instructions can be tape-recorded for private use at home or in the workplace if opportunity occurs. There is little experimentally controlled evidence to support it. However, some comparisons have been made (Turk and Genest 1979; McCauley *et al.* 1983). From a review of twenty-one studies, five of which were controlled, Linton (1982) claimed to have found positive results in terms of reduced pain ratings. This conclusion was confirmed in a later report (Linton 1986), and similar findings have been reported by Turner and Chapman (1982b) and Philips (1988).

However, two recent systematic reviews, covering relaxation with both acute and chronic pain, have produced little evidence to support relaxation in terms of its ability to reduce pain ratings (Seers and Carroll 1998; Carroll and Seers 1998). Rigorous criteria were used, similar to those suggested by Melzack and Wall (1996) to select suitable studies (Jadad *et al.* 1996), involving randomised controlled trials (RCTs). Forty acute studies were identified but of these only seven were eligible for review in meeting the criteria. They utilised a variety of techniques to achieve relaxation, and the definitions and descriptions left much to be desired for comparison. There were also inadequacies in the reporting of pain measures. Of the seven studies included, only four reported statistically significant reductions in pain scores, and one of these was for 'pain distress' rather than a pain score (Seers and Carroll 1998).

Nine studies of relaxation for chronic pain were selected from thirty-two, using the same criteria (Carroll and Seers 1998). Again there was little evidence according to these criteria to support the use of relaxation for the reduction of pain ratings. Only three studies reported statistically significant differences in favour of relaxation. Again there were methodological inadequacies. The authors argue for much improvement in research techniques. However, it might also be suggested that other outcomes could be studied as well, such as a reduction in anxiety, improvement in morale and motivation. There are difficulties in measuring such outcomes but it is not impossible. It could be argued that as a self-administered technique, if it is enjoyed by the patient and provides relief in whatever way, as determined by them, or enables them to cope more effectively with life, then it must be seen as a valuable adjunct to the management of pain.

Biofeedback

This process is a mixture of psychological and physical aspects of pain, and is essentially used as a facilitator of relaxation. It involves the mental control of physiological processes through the mediating effect of feedback. To a certain extent it can be seen as operant conditioning whereby knowledge of results improves performance (Horn and Munafo 1997). The patient receives auditory and/or visual signals about the state of, say, muscular tension, blood pressure, pulse, skin temperature or the galvanic skin response. With more sophisticated systems it might include EEG signals. Turk and

Genest (1979) argue that it works more by cognitive change than physical and recommend using straight cognitive-behavioural approaches. Reviewing an extensive series of studies of the use of biofeedback with a variety of pain problems, Jessup and Gallegos (1994) find that biofeedback and relaxation are well established as treatment interventions, and can be particularly helpful with difficult cases. However, the research evidence to date is rather weak through the use of poorly designed studies. Lack of clarity about the particular intervention, the nature of controls if any, and the lack of definition of the pain syndrome have been identified as areas needing improvement. These are similar problems identified for research into psychological approaches to relaxation above.

Attention and distraction

These two processes are related, in that by paying attention to a stimulus other than the pain, relief might be obtained. There would seem to be a few different types and these have been classified by Melzack and Wall (1996). One type is in fact the focus of attention on the pain itself, known as somatisation. Another is focusing on external events and a third is focusing on internal events to the exclusion of the pain.

Somatisation

This technique involves paying attention to the pain stimulus itself. It involves making a detached analysis of the experience, removal of the emotion, but perhaps acknowledging the presence of emotion and clinically analysing it. It might include ratings and measurement of various aspects of the experience. In this way the pain can be distanced from the individual and come almost to seem that it belongs to someone else.

Distraction

In this procedure, the focus of attention is on events or processes on which concentration is focused. With external stimuli, this might involve the analysis of or involvement in some very intricate process. It may involve timing or counting of steps or phases. Johnson *et al.* (1998) have found that attention to external cues has more impact on pain than using imagery. However, Weisenberg *et al.* (1998) have used films as distractors. They compared humorous, holocaust and neutral films with each other and a no-film group. There were three lengths of film in each group. The results indicated that the humorous film led to an increased pain tolerance as did the longer film in each of the groups. The tolerance test occurred 39 minutes after the films.

With internal stimuli the attention is concentrated inwards to mental processes, such as counting backwards, reciting poetry, or reliving memories. It might involve imagery in that the patient uses images, which may be based on memories to create a mental picture of a pleasant, relaxing situation which can be lived through. All the senses can be involved in the creation of the images, sounds, smells, tastes, to the fullest extent of which the patient is capable. It has been reported as being helpful for patients with cancer, easing pain and anxiety, and enabling them to cope with chemotherapy and other treatments.

The images must be of interest to the patient if guided imagery is being used and therefore the patient must be involved in planning the intervention, or in rehearsing the process. The effort involved must be consistent with the patient's ability to concentrate and be involved physically. Ideally it should start before the pain becomes severe (McCaffrey *et al.* 1994). Some patients develop their own distracting images, and may be ashamed of these. It is important to encourage them and help the patient to use them to maximum effect (Copp 1974).

Music

This can be both internal and external if it involves watching a performance or even participating in a performance. The main effect is from the influence of the music on the thoughts and emotions of the listener (Zimmerman *et al.* 1989; Larson-Beck 1991). Music can have a powerful effect on the emotions but the kinds of music that are likely to have an effect will vary tremendously from individual to individual. A small-scale study by Smith and Noon (1998) has demonstrated the different effects of three types of popular music on moods. They found that dance music had the most positive effect, lifting depression, reducing anxiety and anger, and increasing vigour.

Pain-focused imagery

A specialised use of imagery has been developed (McCaffrey *et al.* 1994), whereby the pain is concentrated on and then imagery is used to create a new image of the pain which can then be controlled and made to flow away from the body.

Cognitive reframing

In this process the pain is re-evaluated together with the pain context and the general lifestyle of the patient. This involves changing the perceptions, understandings and beliefs about pain and the processes associated with pain. In this way a new more positive view of pain and its effect on one's life can be created (Turner and Chapman 1982b; Turk and Rudy 1986). This process is particularly helpful with chronic pain. Specific pain cognitive coping strategies may increase perception of control over pain (Haythornthwaite *et al.* 1998).

Five stages to the process of reframing are suggested, following an individual interview: identifying dysfunctional thoughts and learning to monitor them; recognising the specific connections between emotions, behaviours and thoughts; substituting more positive thoughts; identifying and altering the dysfunctional under-lying beliefs and attitudes; practising coping and modification techniques (Fishman and Loscalzo 1987). Manchini *et al.* (1988) report substantial changes following treatment (see also Williams *et al.* 1993). The process tends also to include relaxation and some researchers argue that it is the relaxation and/or imagery that does the trick (see Horn and Munafo 1997; and see review by Skevington 1995). However, see comments above about the effectiveness of relaxation (Seers and Carroll 1998; Carroll and Seers 1998).

Cognitive-behavioural treatment – operant conditioning

As indicated above, Fordyce (1976) was the first to propose the use of operant strategies in the management of pain and they were developed by others, e.g. Turk *et al.* (1983). However, the programmes nowadays tend to include a range of behaviours including pain, such as some of the concomitants of pain: lack of mobility, reduced activity, low morale, poor sleep and social relationships. The pain behaviours are operants which are reinforced. The treatment involves non-reinforcement of these behaviours and the positive reinforcement of adaptive behaviours. Reinforcers include praise, increased attention or other rewards that have particular meaning for the patient. Turk and Flor (1987) have published a classification of reinforcers: direct positive reinforcers; indirect positive reinforcers; and negative reinforcers (see above). Many programmes will concentrate only on the disabilities rather than the pain itself, to enable the patient to have a more productive life and a better response to pain treatment and ability to cope with it.

A model programme has been developed by Turk and Fernandez (1991) which is multi-dimensional, and includes relaxation and the use of imagery. A recent study by Jensen and Bodin (1998) demonstrated the effectiveness of a multi-modal cognitive-behavioural treatment programme for chronic spinal pain. Another study by LeFort et al. (1998) has recently demonstrated the value of a multi-method psycho-educational programme. This was delivered over a six-week period by community nurses to facilitate the self-management of chronic pain. The course is based on maximum participation and minimum didactic presentation to enable a more individualised approach.

There have been difficulties with research into this kind of intervention, as with other kinds of psychological and also physical treatments – a failure to use control groups being a major weakness (Linton 1982). However, the multi-dimensionality of the programmes makes it difficult to set up controls. Linton reported that there is some evidence of improvement (1982, 1986; and see also Jensen and Bodin 1998). Skevington (1986, 1995) argues that all that happens is that patients learn to be more stoical about their pain, and Pither (1989) claims that that is the aim. The treatment is also costly as it requires hospitalisation for four to six weeks. Because of this others have developed shorter programmes which also include muscular relaxation (for example, Taylor et al. 1980). A recent systematic review and meta-analysis of randomised controlled trials identified twenty-five studies that met the criteria (Morley et al. 1999). It was concluded that cognitive-behavioural treatments significantly reduced behavioural expression of pain, and improved the pain experience, cognitive coping and increased positive appraisal.

These programmes tend to need specialised training and are usually undertaken by psychologists. However, frequently nurses or other professionals are involved, particularly in identifying suitable individual reinforcers, and in applying them. The programme would probably be planned by the psychologist, or someone with special training.

Hypnosis

This technique has been tried with people in pain. However, there is much uncertainty as to exactly what happens during this procedure. Spanos *et al.* (1994) have reviewed the use of hypnosis in laboratory situations and in the clinical field. There is much evidence about its use in the laboratory, although the relevance of these findings to the clinical situation is questioned (e.g. Gauld 1986). However, Spanos *et al.* (1994), as a result of their review, argue that the laboratory findings do generalise well to the clinical setting, although the quality of the studies varied. The authors of the review claim that some of the studies were of good scientific merit but give no details. The conclusions are that hypnotic analgesia treatments are more effective than no treatment in reducing reported pain. Also the results indicate that comparisons between hypnotic and non-hypnotic treatments usually found no difference in therapeutic efficacy. A more recent study by Faymonville *et al.* (1997) demonstrated that hypnosis was better at gaining peri-operative pain and anxiety relief than conventional stress-reducing strategies. It also allowed for significant reductions in medication, improved patient satisfaction and surgical conditions.

A weakness with the clinical studies to date is that they have focused entirely on pain outcome. There is a need, argue Spanos *et al.* (1994), for studies that look also at mediating processes such as coping and compliance phenomena. The issue of hypnotisability has been studied also, and does not seem to be an issue. The patient–therapist relationship seems to be more important (Katz *et al.* 1987). A recent study utilising positron-emission tomography (PET) suggests that hypnosis affects the cortical and subcortical regions of the brain and is likely to be more influential regarding the motivational-emotional and cognitive-evaluative aspects of pain, rather than the sensory-discriminative ones, particularly with reference to the unpleasant aspects of the pain experience (Rainville *et al.* 1997). There is therefore support for the importance of developing psychological strategies to deal with the meanings and emotions associated with persistent pain states.

Information giving

Anxiety has been shown to be a factor in the experience of pain, particularly with acute and post-operative pain (see Chapter 4). Studies have shown that information given before surgery or invasive procedures can reduce anxiety and also influence the pain experience.

There is some uncertainty about the nature of the anxiety effect, as some studies seem to imply that state anxiety is important whereas others that trait anxiety is more important (Weisenberg 1994). Trait anxiety is more of a personality type, whereas state anxiety is that provoked by a particular situation. The evidence suggests that it is the trait anxiety that is more important. Johnson and Vogele (1993) argue nevertheless that attempts to reduce pre-operative anxiety therefore through information giving are most important.

This has been confirmed by some early studies in the UK (Hayward 1975; Boore 1978), as well as in some American ones (Johnson *et al.* 1978). Davis (1984a) found reduction in pain intensity and bearability, as well as an increase in oral non-opioid analgesia given on demand, following information about the sensory experience, the procedures involved and some coping strategies. These latter findings suggest an influence of information on the ability to cope with the pain (its bearability), and increased requests for analgesics by patients when told that they should not wait to be asked or for a particular time period to pass.

A patient education programme, with information about the basic principles of pain and its management, how to use a pain diary, and how to communicate their pain and how to contact health-care workers was developed by de Wit *et al.* (1997) for cancer patients. It produced a reduction in pain ratings and an increase in knowledge. Other studies have demonstrated that people have different styles of coping with stress (e.g. Miller 1988; Gattuso *et al.* 1992), and those who deny stress seem to have a poorer response to information than those who attempt to deal with it (Weisenberg 1994).

Psychological interventions and children

Generally each of the psychological interventions discussed above can be used with children. Relaxation can be used frequently with children, and is perhaps better for relieving distress. Progressive muscle relaxation is also possible with children if they can understand the instructions, and deep breathing can help too (McGrath and de Veber 1986). Special children's programmes have been developed (McGrath *et al.* 1990) and the use of biofeedback recommended (Labbe and Williamson 1984). With very young children and infants, rocking and stroking can help to relax them as can making a 'nest' for them in their bed or cot (D'Apolita 1984; Roop Moyer and Howe 1991).

Distraction can be very effective with children, who seem to find it easy to participate in fantasy to make the pain more bearable (Twycross *et al.* 1998). Types of activity suitable for children include holding and talking about a familiar object or toy; listening to stories or familiar music; singing; solving puzzles (McCaffrey *et al.* 1994). The actual activity used should be chosen with the child and/or parent. The use of imagery can help in that the child can be helped to focus on the pain and imagine it as something else and then imagine it as moving away or getting smaller (Doody *et al.* 1991). The image should incorporate all the senses or as many as possible: visual, auditory, taste, touch and smell (P. A. McGrath 1990).

Cognitive strategies can be used with the older child who can conceptualise his or her pain. Other behavioural approaches can also be used. Exercise and play have an important role (P. A. McGrath 1990) as does reinforcement as part of a structured programme, where meaningful rewards are negotiated with the child and parents and a written contract is agreed (P. A. McGrath 1990). Developing the skill of thought stopping is also of value whereby the child learns particular thoughts or sayings that can be introduced to stop unpleasant thoughts (McGrath *et al.* 1993; Twycross *et al.* 1998).

Hypnosis is recommended for the older child (Carter 1994), who refers to recent research such as Hilgard and LeBaron (1984) for cancer; Olness and Gardner (1988) for relief of distress; Valente (1991) for painful procedures. However, the points made above with regard to the use of hypnosis with adults also apply with children. P. A. McGrath (1990) suggests three uses of hypnosis: the reduction of pain; altering the awareness of the pain; and directing the attention away, citing Hilgard and Hilgard (1983).

Finally, information can play an important role, as with adults. It should be about the sensory experience and the procedures involved. It can involve handling pieces of equipment, practising with a doll, and the discussion of fears, feelings and what is going to happen (Twycross *et al.* 1998). However, with young children it is best if the information is given as close to the event as possible, so that they can remember and link the two together (Weisenberg 1994). The relief of parental anxiety through information giving can also help the child.

Conclusion

The cognitive-evaluative aspects of the pain experience have been shown to be important, and consequently a wide variety of interventions in that domain to help in the management of pain have been developed. Many of the interventions do have a direct effect on the intensity of pain, and lead to reduced pain ratings. However, many of the interventions are focused on the strengthening or development of coping strategies particularly in the chronic pain situation, and have relevance for social aspects of the pain experience.

Psychological approaches are usually seen as adjunctive to pharmacological interventions. They can help to reduce a dependence on medication, and perhaps, rarely, enable someone to do without medication if only for a while. In some chronic and terminal pain situations, pharmacological preparations cannot achieve a satisfactory level of pain control. In such cases the introduction of psychological methods can be very effective. Many of them do require specialist training and sometimes specialist equipment. Nevertheless some of them can be applied by well-prepared health-care professionals, particularly nurses.

Psychological approaches to the management of pain are an important part of the pain armoury, and knowledge about the possibilities should be part of the education and preparation of every nurse specialising in the management of pain.

Part IV

The management of pain

Chapter 9

The assessment and monitoring of pain

Suffering is permanent, obscure and dark,
and shares the nature of infinity

Wordsworth

Introduction

This part of the book is concerned with the management of pain. It is not enough to understand the experience of pain and the mechanisms that bring it about, nor the kinds of interventions that might be brought into play. It is also necessary to have some insight as to the nature of the pain experience in order to select the right form of intervention or interventions. We have therefore to gain some information from the person experiencing the pain in order to be able to help him or her. It is also necessary to have some sort of organisation to co-ordinate the delivery of the pain-management service.

It is only in the light of an understanding of a particular person's individual experience that as effective an intervention as possible might be put into place. We have emphasised the individuality of the pain experience, and also the intrapersonal nature of it. It is known only to the person experiencing it. Without information about the nature of the particular experience we can only guess at it, and thus use standardised approaches to relieve the pain as much as possible and to enable the sufferer to cope as effectively as possible. Unfortunately, guesswork is not a sufficiently accurate foundation on which to base health-care interventions. Standardised approaches help the average person but not any particular person. No one is average when it comes to illness, in particular with respect to pain, although evidence quoted in the first chapter indicates that this tends to be the approach being used in too many instances.

In this chapter, we shall be looking at the relationship of the assessment of pain to the information considered in Parts II and III. In these we have discussed the sensory-discriminative, motivational-emotional and cognitive-evaluative aspects of the pain experience and the various kinds of interventions that are now available to help to relieve or reduce pain, and to help the person in pain cope with the pain experience. The kinds of assessments that we might undertake reflect the various aspects of the nature of the pain experience, as well as what it is possible to do about it. Following on this preparatory discussion the various forms and processes of assessment will be presented and reviewed. Finally there is a special section on the assessment of pain in children and infants.

Why assess pain?

As indicated above the determination as to which interventions and at what intensity to prescribe and administer them to someone in pain is difficult if there has been no assessment of the nature of the pain experience. There is much evidence that this is one of the weakest aspects of the management of pain (Zalon 1993), and yet one aspect that seems to be particularly suited to the role of the nurse (Seers 1987; Carr 1997). A most important principle is of course that we have to depend largely on information from the person themselves. There is some information that can be used from physiological and behavioural sources, but there are many limitations to this kind of information, which we shall discuss in due course.

There are many instruments and procedures now available to help the nurse or indeed any other professional to assess pain, and we shall be looking at these in some detail. However, first it is important to consider the nature of the information that will be helpful in making decisions about interventions. As indicated in Box 6.2 on p. 103 (based on the work of the WHO (1980), Kleinman (1988), and Helman (1994)), there are different aspects to disease at the biological, the psychological and the social levels or planes. The practitioners tend to take a biological view of signs in determining the presence of a health-care problem; the patient takes more of a bio-psychological view of symptoms in determining the presence of a health-care problem; and society takes more of a social view in terms of the effect of the health-care problem on the ability of the patient to play her or his various roles in society as being what is known as sickness or disability. The implication is that the assessments should explore these different planes or aspects of the experience. As discussed in Chapter 6, in many ways these planes echo the four aspects that we have been studying: the sensory-discriminative, the motivational-emotional, the cognitive-evaluative and the social and cultural.

What sort of information will be helpful?

Figure 9.1 indicates the range of signs and symptoms that can be used in an assessment. In general as thorough an assessment as possible should be made to ensure that all aspects are dealt with when planning care. However, sometimes, particularly in the acute or emergency situation, there is no time. McCaffrey *et al.* (1994) have recognised this and offer a simple short assessment procedure to enable some intervention to be planned in relation to that particular person's pain. In this they suggest that the site of the pain, the mobility and duration of the pain, a verbal rating of the pain on a 1–10 scale and indication of any medication being taken at the time, and its efficacy, should provide enough information to enable interventions to be planned and prescribed in the short term. A more full assessment can then be made as time allows.

Instrumentation

A wide variety of instruments have been developed in order to collect information from people in pain. Some are quite sophisticated and probably more suitable for research purposes as they collect a lot of specialised information to test out the hypotheses of the research. Generally the simpler forms of assessment are more suitable for clinical application. Nevertheless the same principles of rigour should apply to the collection of clinical data as to the collection of research data.

These principles include validity, reliability, versatility and bias. P. A. McGrath (1990) has discussed these issues with particular reference to the assessment of pain in children. However, the same principles apply to the assessment of pain in adults. With regard to validity, it must be clear what exactly is being measured by the instrument. Is it the intensity, duration, bearability or is it the

Signs

Any behavioural aspects	*or physiological aspects*
Holding	Raised pulse rate
Guarding	Raised respiration
Withdrawing	Shock
Crying	Inflammation
Grimacing	

Symptoms

Sensory-discriminative symptoms	*Emotional-motivational aspects*
The site or location of the pain	Anxiety and stress
The intensity of the pain	Changes in mood
The pattern or frequency of the pain	Coping ability
The duration of the pain	*Cognitive-evaluative aspects*
The presence of any other associated symptoms	The quality of the pain, what it feels like
The effect of any intervention	The meaning of the pain experience for the person

Socio-cultural aspects

Any psycho-social factors of the pain experience

The factors or situations that increase or aggravate the pain

Figure 9.1   Signs and symptoms for pain assessment

emotional aspects of the pain experience? Reliability means that the instrument must give the same reading on different occasions if the experience is unchanged. Alternatively it must accurately record changes in the experience. The instrument must not be influenced by any biases in the observer or the person experiencing the pain. Thus attitudes or prejudices must not be able to be expressed or reported on the instrument. Finally the instrument should be as versatile as possible, that is not too dependent on a particular pain situation.

P. A. McGrath (1990) also makes a point about the kind of data collected by instruments. This affects what can be done with the data. Four types of data are acknowledged: nominal, ordinal, interval and ratio. Nominal data consists of types, classes or categories of information. Verbal information describing the pain experience can be dealt with as nominal, in that the words used can be classified. Some scales have been developed with groups of words already classified, for example the McGill Pain Questionnaire (Melzack 1975). Ordinal data is that which indicates more or less of a particular attribute, but no particular amount. It is possible to rank order things, for example the pain may be more intense or less intense than previously, without a particular numerical score or rating being applied. Some verbal rating scales are of this kind whereby the words describing more or less pain do not indicate any particular amount or quantity. The faces scales used in the assessment of pain in children are also of this kind. Although frequently used in association with a numerical scale there is little evidence to indicate that there is a good correlation between the numerical scale and the ordinal faces scale.

If it is necessary to indicate how much more or less the pain, then one moves into the interval or ratio data set. Interval data is frequently collected for pain assessment with numerical rating scales which have fixed intervals. The assumption is that each interval is of equal value, thus the increase from one to two is the same as that from two to three and so on. The person being assessed indicates which number on the scale best represents the amount of pain experienced. There are problems with allocating numbers to a verbal rating scale. The 'distance' or interval between the meanings of the various words on the scale may not be equal as is assumed with a straight numerical scale.

The ratio scale is the most accurate and offers the most facility in mathematical and statistical manipulation. Frequently the person is asked to indicate where along a line ranging from no pain to the worst possible pain, their pain is. This gives a length of line or distance from no pain to the point indicated by the person in pain. This distance can be measured with great accuracy to decimal points. It is this kind of data that can produce mean pain scores for example. The mode would be the most suitable way of similarly handling the other kinds of data, being the most frequently occurring score, words or class of words. The median is useful if there is a suitably wide range of scores, being the central score in a rank-ordered range of scores.

Behavioural and physiological assessment of pain

These methods are of particular value when it is difficult or impossible for the person in pain to give verbal or written indication of the nature of their pain. Such situations may occur with the elderly, with people with learning difficulties or mental illness, where there are language problems, with young children, or when the person is very shocked.

The behavioural indicators include sounds such as cries and whimpers or expressions of anger or other negative changes of mood; facial expressions or tears; and movements of the limbs and body. There may be guarding of parts of the body, or lack of movement, as in a stiffening of a part of the body and a resistance to movement. The person may seem to be in an uncomfortable or unusual position. There is always the problem of interpretation here, and care must be taken. In the presence of signs of injury or potential injury or disease, then, such signs can be useful indicators. There is little to be lost in assuming pain and providing an intervention. If the intervention changes the behaviour for the better then this can act as confirmation.

There have been attempts to catalogue facial expressions and other behaviours in young infants. These will be discussed in more detail in that section.

Physiological signs are more difficult to interpret as many of them can have different causes. Nevertheless most of the signs that can be of value relate to changes in the sympathetic nervous system, indicating stress and a response to it. As we have seen in Chapter 2 on the sensory-discriminative aspects of pain, this system is frequently involved in the pain experience. Thus the physiological signs can support other indicators, and might include heart rate, blood pressure and sweating. Such measures may already be being taken as part of general observation of a person in pain, injured or as part of pre- or post-operative care.

Sensory-discriminative assessment of pain

The site or location of the pain can be identified by the person pointing to or touching the part of the body concerned. There may be more than one site of pain, if there are multiple injuries or surgical interventions, or with some disease processes causing pain, as in arthritis, or cancer. A body chart can be useful, such as that forming part of the McGill Pain Questionnaire (see Figure 9.3 below). Other charts include details of the sides of the body as well as the front and back, and also head and feet in larger scale (for example in the Initial Pain Assessment Tool of McCaffrey *et al.* (1994)). The nurse or the person in pain may make the mark or marks to indicate the location of the pain. The amount of detail required will depend on the general purposes of the assessment and the nature of the pain. The total area covered by the pain can be indicated by shading or colouring in the area. The Oxford Pain Relief Unit Body Chart uses a body chart which also includes the dermatomes which reflect the sensory enervation of the body (see Carroll 1993 for an example and Chapter 2). This can be very helpful when attempting to diagnose the cause of the pain or to understand referred pain situations.

The intensity of the pain will be of most importance to the person in pain and it is of course important to the nurse or other health-care professional involved. Most interventions will be aimed at reducing intensity and so an accurate estimation of that is very important. Rating scales are the most common, either verbal or numerical scales. Various ranges of numbers can be used, such as 0–5; 0–10; or 0–100. Usually 0 means no pain and the highest number on the scale means the worst possible pain. Some scales do not have numbers written on them, but merely consist of a line of say 100 mm length which can then be measured once the person has indicated with a mark along the line how much above '0' or no pain is their pain at present to give a score or rating out of 100 (see Figure 9.2). The scales may be horizontal or vertical. If vertical they may be called pain thermometers by some. They are usually known collectively as Visual Analogue Scales (VAS).

A VAS may be used to measure the maximum level of pain that can be tolerated before an intervention is called for, as part of the management programme. The author has used a numerical VAS to rate the bearability of the pain, as a different but complementary indicator from intensity. An intervention may make the pain more bearable but not necessarily make a significant difference to the intensity (Davis 1984a; and Figure 9.3). The interventions may be psycho-social in nature and thus this measure may be useful in assessing the effect of coping strategies.

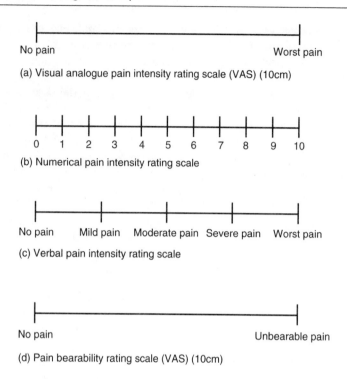

Figure 9.2 Pain rating scales

Verbal indicators are more problematic, in that the interpretation of the verbal indicator may not be consistent, even with the same person on different occasions, as they gain more experience of their pain. Terms such as 'a little pain', 'a moderate amount of pain', or 'a lot of pain' can be helpful initially but are not very helpful in assessing the effect of any intervention. The verbal 'steps' on the scale may sometimes be converted to numbers and thus used as a numerical scale.

The pattern or frequency of the pain can provide important information in aiding diagnosis, as also may the presence of any other associated symptoms. This information is usually collected verbally as part of an assessment interview. Certain disease processes, such as cardiovascular disorders, and some rheumatic conditions present identifiable pain pictures. Then pain may remit and then return in association with other factors such as movement or exercise, or high levels of anxiety or stress. Some headaches are of this kind, as also are certain facial pains. The pain may be sustained at a fairly even level, but with occasional superimposed paroxysms.

The pattern and frequency of the pain are also associated with the duration of the pain. The timescale of any patterns or rates of the pain experience should be recorded. This may be in terms of minutes, hours or even days and weeks. In the case of chronic pain it is very important to record the length of time the person has been in pain. Chronicity is determined to a certain extent by time, and a usual figure for pain to be considered chronic is three months; however, it is also defined as being pain that persists after healing has occurred or long after it can have served any useful function (Bonica 1974; Melzack and Wall 1996). Duration may be important regarding diagnosis of the underlying problem.

It is very important to record the effect of any intervention. This information can usually be obtained from the person in pain, and some of the scales discussed above may be used in this process. However, there may be other aspects than the intensity or bearability of the pain that might need to be recorded. In assessing the pain experience any factors or functions influenced by the pain should be considered in evaluating the outcomes of interventions, and these will be considered when we look at the motivational-emotional, cognitive-evaluative, and social and cultural aspects.

Motivational-emotional assessment of pain

Anxiety

Anxiety and stress are frequent concomitants of pain or of the anticipation of pain. There are scales available for the assessment of levels of anxiety and stress, some of which are suitable for clinical application (e.g. Spielberger *et al.* 1970, 1983). If there are concerns that anxiety is approaching a debilitating level warranting medical intervention, then a validated test should be used. However, this kind of determination of anxiety is more frequently used in research settings. There are approaches which can help the person in pain or the person anticipating pain to express anxieties in a conversational, verbal style. Asking the person what their expectations are of the situation can stimulate the expression of any fears or anxieties.

Anxiety is usually associated with uncertainty or ignorance about procedures or their outcome. People can have very strong fears and worries about coming into hospital and undergoing invasive treatments or surgery (Davis 1984b). Often the process of assessing any such fears or worries can be linked directly with information giving which can then act to relieve the uncertainty. This may apply to the pre-operative situation or to a situation after injury where a person with pain is to undergo some movement or investigation, or with the person with chronic pain undergoing investigation or interventions.

Depression and other mood changes

Changes in mood can also be assessed. Depression is not infrequently associated with chronic pain for example. Anger and frustration can also be experienced by the sufferer and information about these emotional effects of the pain experience should be collected so that they can be incorporated in the plan of care. There are validated instruments for the assessment of depression (such as the Beck scale – Beck *et al.* 1988), and they should be used if there is concern as to the level of depression being experienced by the person in pain. If the changes in mood do warrant medical intervention then the validated instruments might be useful in assessing the effectiveness of any intervention. However, clinical signs and symptoms expressed are usually enough.

A conversational-style interview can elicit information about changes in mood which can inform interventions. This may be associated with collecting information about the meaning of the pain for the person; often the meaning involves the emotional connotations as well as any others. Information about anger and frustration can be collected in a similar way through interview and it may similarly be associated with the meaning of the pain or the effect of the pain on social activities or roles.

Coping

The ability or willingness of the person in pain or who is anticipating pain to participate in, comply with, or initiate coping strategies must also be assessed. Often the efficacy of an intervention depends on the willingness of the person in pain to undergo tiresome or painful procedures to try to improve things. A not uncommon experience is that of feelings of helplessness or hopelessness in the chronic pain situation. These may also be associated with feelings of depression. Similarly a sense of losing control or of getting out of control of oneself and one's abilities and roles can be experienced by the person in pain. McCracken (1998) argues that acceptance of the pain leads to reports of lower pain intensity, less pain-related anxiety, less depression, less physical and psycho-social disability, more daily up time, and better work status.

There are coping scales and measures of sense of control (e.g. the Coping Strategy Questionnaire, Rosensteil and Keefe 1983; Beliefs in Pain Control Questionnaire, Skevington 1990). Haythornthwaite *et al.* (1998) found positive outcomes correlated with perceptions of control over pain, and in particular, the use of specific cognitive pain-coping strategies facilitated this. Also, using the Pain Beliefs and Perceptions Inventory (PBPI), Williams *et al.* (1994) demonstrated that when pain becomes persistent, patients may change their previously held cultural or personal beliefs about pain, and form new ones. Nevertheless these are usually used in the research setting but can be used in the clinical situation if there is concern that these feelings are very detrimental to the progress of any treatment, although Morley and Wilkinson (1995) have reservations about the clinical use of the PBPI.

The interview as a form of information collection is perhaps to be preferred in the clinical situation when the issues can be explored in some detail and the personal, individual aspects can be picked up. There are also links between emotion, motivation, and coping with the meaning of the pain, and in an interview all of these aspects can be explored together. Certainly feelings of helplessness or hopelessness can be identified more effectively in this way. This is discussed more in the next section.

Cognitive-evaluative assessment of pain

The quality of the pain

The quality of the pain, what it feels like to the person experiencing it, can be of great importance to the people trying to help relieve the pain or to help the person to cope with the pain. The person can be asked to describe in their own words what the pain is like. Alternatively they can be asked to indicate on a list of words which of them most aptly describe their experience. The McGill Pain Questionnaire contains such a list divided into different categories (Melzack 1975, 1983; and Figure 9.3). This was developed from a study of the language of pain (Melzack and Torgerson 1971). The words were derived from the clinical literature concerning people in pain and also from some interviews with people in pain. The study demonstrated a great deal of agreement as to the use of the words in describing pain. The instrument lists 78 adjectives reflecting the sensory, cognitive-evaluative and the emotional aspects of the pain experience, as well as some miscellaneous words that seem to be used frequently by people in pain. The scale is scored by counting the number of words in each of the categories and also the total number of words.

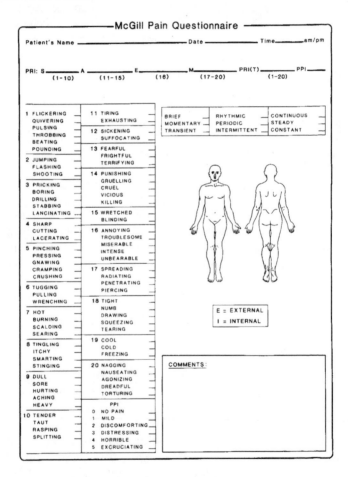

Figure 9.3   The McGill Pain Questionnaire

Source: © Robert Melzack, reprinted with permission

There are criticisms of the instrument, in that the words are imposed on the person rather than them choosing their own. There is also the problem of cultural factors influencing the use of words, although there are now several versions of the instrument in other languages (see Melzack and Katz 1992; Kim *et al.* 1995). Skevington (1995) has offered a substantial critique of the questionnaire, and points out the failure to allow people in pain to confirm the validity of the categories of pain or even of the words used. Some words do seem to be those used by professionals rather than ordinary people in pain. Nevertheless it continues to be one of the most frequently used instruments, in both clinical and research settings. Because it is rather time consuming, a shortened version has been developed which is perhaps more suitable for the acute or emergency setting (Melzack 1987).

Self-esteem

The self-esteem of a person in pain is an important indicator as is the sense of being in control, or at the mercy of others. There are instruments to assess these aspects of the experience (e.g. Rotter 1966 for locus of control, and Coopersmith 1981 for self-esteem). Again they tend to be used more in the research setting but can be useful in making a thorough assessment, particularly in the chronic pain situation where the impact of these factors can be very strong. Self-esteem can be valuable as there are interventions aimed at strengthening it and a measure to assess the effectiveness of the intervention is useful. Low self-esteem can also be seen as associated with feelings of helplessness and depression, and the assessment of these could usefully go together.

The meaning of the pain

The meaning of the pain experience for the person can also be obtained through interview and this is a recommended procedure (McCaffrey *et al.* 1994). However, this can also be a time consuming exercise and is perhaps more suitable in the chronic pain situation when a thorough assessment of motivational-emotional, cognitive-evaluative, and psycho-social aspects mentioned above are more important. During an interview the collection of information using rating scales or tests can be undertaken as well.

The meaning of the pain in a terminal situation or where the prognosis is very poor, as with cancer for example, can be very important in determining the approach to care. The meaning may change over time or as the disease progresses. The collection of information about the meaning of the pain should be a continuing process with discussions or conversations with the person in pain occurring periodically in order to monitor this aspect. This would apply to all chronic situations.

Pain diaries

One way of maintaining a picture of the developing and changing pain situation is for the person to keep a diary of their pain experience. These can be very valuable in a retrospective analysis of the effectiveness or otherwise of any interventions. It can also act as a warning of the development of any emotional or social problems. People in pain can find the very process of keeping this record of their thoughts and feelings, their experiences and reactions to events, including therapeutic events, a very rewarding experience, particularly with children (Carter 1994). It can help them to cope with the situation and reflect on it. A variety of formats for such diaries have been developed, but many people develop their own (see McCaffrey *et al.* 1994). A particular kind of diary suitable for use in the home by chronic cancer pain patients has been devised by de Wit *et al.* (1999) and evaluated in The Netherlands.

Socio-cultural assessment of pain

Any socio-cultural factors of the pain experience, particularly in the chronic pain situation, can also be explored through an interview, or through a diary. There are also some questionnaires which have been developed to explore family relationships and work roles (e.g. Epstein and Bishop 1981; Olson *et al.* 1984; see also Roy 1992). However, as with some other instruments these can be time consuming to use and are more frequently used for research purposes rather than in the clinical situation. If there are cultural issues to be explored to determine the meaning of the pain and its effect on the person's response to the pain or compliance with therapy then the interview will be a necessary procedure with, perhaps, the help of others from the particular culture or a translator. The others here might include members of the family, or senior members of the local cultural group. The organisation of such interviews including others will be discussed further in Chapter 10, when we consider management issues.

Assessment of the family relationships, the kind of work, and social activities carried out by the person should be explored at interview, and the effect of the pain on them assessed. Issues to be considered include the effects on the family, in particular on the spouse or partner, and the role relationships within the partnership. If the 'family' involves a very elderly parent and an elderly son or daughter then the role relationships may also be affected. There may be financial issues to consider as well and referral on to other agencies may be necessary. The work situation can be explored as roles in that setting may be affected too. The work undertaken by the person may have to be changed, or work may no longer be possible and unemployment may loom or have occurred. The individual may have a variety of roles in the local community which mean much to them in terms of their self-identity, self-esteem and sense of importance. Withdrawal from social life can have a very negative effect on the ability or willingness to cope with the pain (Roy 1992).

The activities, factors or situations that increase or aggravate the pain should be assessed also, as part of the review of the effects of the pain on the person's life. Therapeutic interventions can then be aimed at improving the ability of the individual to cope with restricted mobility or other aspects of functioning as well as relief of the pain. The therapeutic interventions may include changes to or developments in the various roles and activities undertaken by the individual. It may be that the partner or other family members may need to be involved in the assessment and the planning, so that a comprehensive picture can be obtained, and a more effective plan of care can then be developed.

The assessment of pain in infants and children

There are particular problems with the assessment of pain in children. McCaffrey *et al.* (1994) argue that the assessment should start with the parents and the child before the pain occurs if possible. This applies obviously in the surgical setting, but is not possible in the accident and emergency setting or with chronic pain. It can happen however when painful interventions are going to occur. The parents should be involved at whatever stage.

Communication skills are at a premium with the management of pain in children and this applies to communication with parents as well as the child. Adaptability is important in order to deal with the differing cognitive levels in children as well as the concerns of the child and those of the parent which might be quite different. In most cases much of the interaction will be with the parents unless the child is relatively mature and verbally articulate. This could occur in the teens or even a little earlier. However, even then it is important to have a parent present in order that as full a picture is obtained as possible, and also to ensure that the child's rights are fully considered, and not ignored under organisational pressure.

Interviews

P. J. McGrath (1990) argues that it is through an interview with the child and perhaps also the parent, that the most valuable information can be gained. There are several issues that should be addressed in an interview with parents of a child in pain or one who is about to be in pain (Carter 1994; Twycross *et al.* 1998). They include the parents' perception of the priorities of the situation, and clarification of their meaning of the word 'pain' with children. It is through discussing these issues that any socio-cultural aspects can be identified and dealt with. Other aspects to be covered in the interview include the child's previous experiences of pain if any; how the parents assess the child's pain; and the importance of telling the team if they think the child is hurting. It is important also to ask the parent how they feel about staying with the child while he/she is in pain; what they usually do to comfort the child or to relieve pain; and their interest or willingness to learn about alternative or complementary methods of managing pain. The parents also need to be informed as to how the various pain-assessment charts, proformas and so on work, and their potential role in completing them.

The child should be included in the interview if possible. If discussing the situation with the child then it is most important that they are made to feel comfortable and relaxed. The language used should not be too sophisticated, and may involve references to toys or dolls in order to explain things or to make a point. It may be possible to touch the child or hold their hand or share a toy with them. It is most important to be honest about pain but not to over-dramatise it at the same time. The child should be given as much opportunity as possible to express him or herself in their own language. It can be helpful for them to use dolls or drawings to tell their story. Do not treat the child 'childishly'. McCaffrey *et al.* (1994) have produced a Parent Interview Questionnaire which incorporates the above points (pp. 232–233).

The main problem with children is the range of verbal and cognitive ability that can be shown with an age range from birth to late teens. The same range of issues about the experience of pain need to be addressed. The older the child the more likely is it that issues of meaning and socio-cultural aspects will be expressed by the child. However, with the infant these issues may be relevant and expressed by or gained from the parent. Generally the assessment of pain in children is divided into two groups, infants (say 0–5 yrs) and children (5 yrs–teens). This reflects the issues about cognitive development considered in Chapter 5, and in particular the development of language.

The ability to communicate pain develops over the months and years of development. For example, from birth to three months it is essentially non-verbal movements and behaviours including crying and facial expression (D'Apolita 1984). From three to six months there is localisation of pain, pointing and holding (Hazinski 1984). From six to eighteen months there seems to be memory of pain, anxiety and fear of a pain stimulus (Levy 1960). From eighteen months to four years there is guarding, bending knees, resting feet on the bed, touching the site, and grimacing (Taylor 1983).

As the child develops, for example as proposed through the Piagetian stages, there is a correlating development of sophistication in expression of pain. This is not necessarily age related (Savendra *et al.* 1982). There are four such stages: the egocentric, the pre-operational, the concrete operational, and the abstract operational. In the egocentric stage there are just the non-verbal expressions of pain. In the pre-operational stage there is the beginning of verbal expression with black and white judgements of good and bad and also feelings of guilt and fear. In the concrete operational stage the verbal development allows expressions of pain such as 'my tummy hurts', 'my head hurts', 'it hurts here' – pointing. In the abstract operational stage there is the ability to see relationships between experiences and events. It is possible to anticipate in the abstract to plan coping strategies and to use analogies and similes to describe the pain. The vocabulary becomes much more rich.

Assessment of pain in infants

The main issue here is the general inability of the infant to express themselves verbally as to their pain experience. There may be sounds as in crying, screaming, or moaning which can give information. The main kinds of information to be gained from the infant are non-verbal, and include physiological, behavioural aspects (both body movements and facial expressions) and sounds. However, these indicators are always potential indicators of other processes. It is important that the possibility of pain as a factor is not forgotten in interpreting these signs. Also it is important to remember that if there are interventions or health problems in the infant, that in an adult would cause pain, then it is likely that pain will be being experienced by the infant. Measures must be taken to reduce the pain, either in advance through skin preparation, or systemically (see the discussion on treatment of pain in infants in Chapter 7). A close observation of the signs described below will help in such a decision.

If there are signs of injury or there has been surgery then, of course, pain will be being experienced and there should be a plan of care incorporating relief of such pain. As indicated in earlier chapters there is strong evidence that the infant can experience pain and we must assume that it is being experienced. Surgery should of course be carried out under anaesthetic. Much of the research into crying and pain has been done during unanaesthetised surgery for circumcision (for example, Porter *et al.* 1986; Fuller *et al.* 1994). It is appalling that still today surgery on infants such as circumcision in boys is carried out without anaesthetic. The surgeons should experience circumcision or other minor surgery themselves without anaesthetic. Their cries might show interesting characteristics as well and produce a useful scale. It would be interesting to see whether or nor they would just get over it as they seem to expect the infant to.

Physiological measures

As with adults the use of physiological measures are limited in the clinical situation, but are frequently used in research. However, with the neonate and very young infant there may very well be ongoing physiological monitoring of the baby's health status and thus the information can be used as part of the clinical decision-making process. The heart rate and respiratory rate are two common indicators monitored and can give evidence of distress if they increase in association with situations that could provoke a pain response. Palmar sweating is another measure used as a sign of stress and if associated with a painful situation could be used. Also cortisol/cortisone levels and transcutaneous oxygen are used in research but require time-consuming processes and are not really suitable for making immediate decisions. It can be argued that they measure distress rather than pain, but as pain causes stress and distress and if the situation suggests that pain might be a part of the distress situation then the assessment should include that possibility and so determine the treatment.

Behavioural measures

More useful indicators that can be assessed are the behavioural ones. Body movements are often much more easy to interpret in relation to what is happening to the infant. Withdrawal of a limb or attempted withdrawal or tension in the limb when a painful intervention is to take place indicates anticipated pain. Similarly such withdrawal on the intervention would indicate pain. Restlessness, or writhing movements or unnatural stillness or stiffness on attempting to move the infant suggest pain or much discomfort. Such movements may be quite large and include flailing of limbs, particularly with an older baby, in attempts to avoid interventions. With an even older infant, there may be guarding of parts of the body or attempts to point to a sore or hurting place.

Facial expressions are also very informative in terms of the infant's emotional state. There has been described a 'pain face' based on videotaped expressions in response to heel lancing (Grunau and Craig 1987; and see Figure 9.4). A Neonatal Facial Coding Scale has been developed from this source (Grunau and Craig 1990). Its use at the bedside in day-to-day clinical use was demonstrated by Grunau et al. (1998). A similar neonatal pain-assessment tool has been developed by Lawrence et al. (1993). Hadjistavropoulos et al. (1997) have demonstrated the value of using facial and behaviour expression in the assessment of pain in pre-term and full-term infants. More elaborate ranges of facial expression have been devised for use with older children (see below).

Crying is also an important indicator of distress. Attempts have been made to identify the characteristics of a 'pain cry', for example Grunau and Craig (1987) and Johnston and Strada (1986). Intensity,

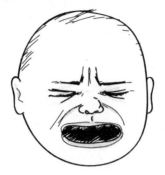

Figure 9.4   The infant 'pain' face

latency and duration seem to be the important factors. As noted above, research undertaken during unanaesthetised circumcision operations indicates that the cry can vary at different stages of the surgery (Porter *et al.* 1986). There is conflicting evidence about the ability of parents to identify a pain cry (for example Murry *et al.* 1977; Petrovitch-Bartell *et al.* 1982).

Nevertheless with contextual clues, body movements, facial expressions and cries there is usually much information available to determine the presence of stress and the likelihood of pain being a factor in that stress. Perhaps the best known multi-dimensional behavioural instrument utilising body and limb movements, facial, verbal, tactile and crying signs of pain is that known as the CHEOPS (the Children's Hospital of East Ontario Pain Scale, McGrath *et al.* 1985). However, it has been noted that it is perhaps measuring distress rather than just pain (McGrath 1989). It has been shown not to be responsive to pain outside the immediate post-operative period (Beyer *et al.* 1990).

Assessment of pain in children

If the child is old enough to be able to express him or herself about the nature of their pain, its intensity, location, meaning and so on then there are a wide variety of methods of collecting such information, as there are with adults. Physiological and behavioural measures are available as with infants but because it is possible to obtain verbal and numerical measures with the older child the nurse or health-care professional is not so dependent on such sources.

They are often used in research however, as they might also be with adults.

Verbal reports

The simplest method is of course to ask the child direct questions if this is possible. In the acute and emergency setting this may be all there is time to do, and the McCaffrey *et al.* (1994) Initial Pain Assessment Tool can also be useful in gaining some initial information on which to base the beginnings of a care plan. Interviews as described above are an important part of the pain-assessment armoury and the various instruments and methods discussed below should be used as part of an interview process. The types of question asked are important. There are different outcomes from open and closed questions, for example, and from structured and semi-structured formats, as in the Children's Comprehensive Pain Questionnaire (P. A. McGrath 1990). This is useful particularly with recurrent and chronic pain in children 5 to 17 years old.

Diaries have been used with some success in an attempt to get a picture of the pain experience over time and perhaps responses to interventions, recording pain ratings together with comments about other symptoms, or aspects of the experience (for example McGrath *et al.* 1990). Gill *et al.* (1997) describe the development of the Central Middlesex Hospital Children's Health Diary (CMHCHD). It is claimed to have potential for clinical and research use particularly for children with sickle cell disease.

Visual Analogue Scales

Generally however attempts are made to gain information in a more structured and formalised way as part of an ongoing care plan. Self-report measures are now used, although their use could be increased. Measures similar to those used with adults can also be used with children, such as visual analogue scales or adjective descriptors such as the McGill. VAS consisting of lines with end points can be used from 5 years onwards and have been shown to correlate with parents' and nurses' ratings (Varni *et al.* 1987). Verbal rating scales may not be so effective. The adjective descriptors are useful with adolescents or even younger (see Gaffney 1988; Abu-Saad 1990). A new analogue scale for assessing children's pain has been developed by McGrath *et al.* (1996), which seems to be of better value clinically than the VAS. It incorporates both colours and faces with numerical ratings. Further work is needed however.

Colour scales

A colour scale has been developed over the years (Eland 1974, 1981, 1985, 1988) which is very effective in helping children to describe their pain and is thought to be useful for 4 to 10 year olds. The child decides which colours mean what degree of pain and then use those colours to indicate on a body chart where their pain is. Black and red seem to be the colours used most frequently to indicate much pain (Eland 1974; Unruh et al. 1983). Poker chips have also been used, typically where the child is asked to indicate with four or five chips how intense their pain is (Hester 1979). It is recommended that this tool is used with 4 to 8 year olds, and that it correlates well with patient and nurse ratings (Hester et al. 1990).

Faces rating scales

Various faces rating scales have been developed. The Oucher Scale (Beyer 1984), the Wong and Baker Scale (1988), and the Bieri et al. Scale (1990) are common examples. The Oucher Scale consists of six faces aligned with a numerical scale of 0–100. It is said to have content validity (Aradine et al. 1987), and ethnic versions have been developed (Beyer et al. 1992). It is claimed to be useful for three to twelve year olds. The Wong and Baker Scale has been shown to be popular with all ages up to 18 years, and consists of six faces. The main criticism of these scales is the possible confusion between pain and happiness–sadness, as the extreme faces at the ends of the scales do seem to represent the latter rather than the face of someone in pain or relaxed and comfortable. The Bieri et al. Scale of seven faces has been developed from drawings by children and does not show laughing or crying but a relaxed face and a 'pain' face (see Figure 9.5) at the extremities of the scale. It is claimed that this makes it a more valid scale (Bieri et al. 1990).

Wong and Baker (1988) have compared six pain-assessment scales: the simple description (verbal) scale; the VAS (1–10); the faces scale; the glasses scale; the poker chips scale; and the colours scale. The faces scale was shown to be the most preferred by children of ages 3–18, but no scale demonstrated superiority with regard to validity or reliability. There was lack of agreement with previous research

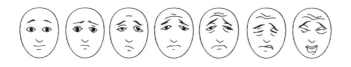

Figure 9.5 Bieri's 'faces' pain rating scale

Source: Reprinted from *Pain* 41, Bieri *et al.*, 'The Faces Pain Scale for the self assessment of the severity of the pain experienced by children: development, initial validation and preliminary investigation for ratio scale properties', pp. 139–50, © 1990, with permission from Elsevier Science

regarding the colour chosen for most pain, least pain and favourite colour. There is obviously much individuality in choice of colour to represent pain in children. It was noted that colour blindness in boys may cause problems and the young children (3 years) could not name the colours.

Generally a holistic approach is recommended (Carter 1994; P. A. McGrath 1990), and there are now multi-dimensional approaches that would seem to offer a more thorough assessment. For example, a Pediatric Pain Questionnaire has been developed by Varni *et al.* (1987), and an Adolescent Pediatric Pain Tool has been developed by Savendra *et al.* (1993). These are multi-dimensional and include verbal descriptors as well as body outlines for location. A Pain Coping Questionnaire for children and adolescents has been developed by Reid *et al.* (1998). It consists of three higher-order scales (approach, problem-focused avoidance, emotion-focused avoidance) and eight sub-scales (information seeking, problem solving, seeking social support, positive self-statements, behavioural distraction, cognitive distraction, externalising and internalising/catastrophising). It is claimed that it can be administered to children of 8 years and older.

It is important to try to obtain sensory, emotional and cognitive-evaluative information in order to gain as good a picture of the pain experience as possible. Also regular routine measurement is important, leading to better pain control (Stevens 1990). Setting the various instruments and assessment procedures in a semi-structured interview setting seems to offer the best opportunity, particularly if the parents can also be present. This process will also ensure the establishment of a more therapeutic relationship with both child and parent.

Conclusion

The assessment of pain is a 'sine qua non' in the management of pain. For both adults and children there are problems in any outsider gaining access to the inside story of the experience of pain. It is important that the professional team gains information about all the possible aspects of the experience described in the first six chapters of this volume, particularly the sensory-discriminative, the motivational-emotional, the cognitive-evaluative, and the socio-cultural. With this information a plan of care can be developed which should then ensure that all aspects of the pain experience are covered. The range of assessment strategies described in this chapter should enable an individual picture of the experience of each person in pain to be gained, and from that an individual programme of care and a suitable range of interventions to be generated. The utilisation of the various interventions, pharmaco-logical, physical or psychological, as are discussed in Chapters 7 and 8, can then be managed by the pain team. The roles of the different professionals and the organisation of interventions in the management of pain are included in the topics of the next chapter.

Chapter 10

Administration of interventions

and relieved their pain …
Goldsmith

Introduction

In the second chapter in this part, we shall be looking at the organisational aspects of the delivery of a service to manage pain, in the acute as well as the chronic situation. This will involve ethical aspects of the management of pain, and the roles played by various professionals, and in particular nurses. It will also involve the way in which these roles are organised, and the relationships between them. We shall look at special situations, such as the management of pain in children, particularly neonates and infants as well as the elderly. Other areas included in this chapter will be the management of cancer pain, and terminal care.

In the introductory chapter the question of poor management of pain was raised, with reference to evidence of the existence of unrelieved or inadequately relieved pain. This referred to the acute or post-operative situation for example (Royal Colleges 1990; Alleyne and Thomas 1994; Melzack *et al.* 1987; Cousins 1994). Reference was also made to the care of children (for example Schechter *et al.* 1986; P. A. McGrath 1990; Cummings *et al.* 1996), to cancer pain and chronic non-malignant pain (Cherny and Portenoy 1994; McCaffrey *et al.* 1994; Richardson 1997). The focus of this volume has been to demonstrate the factors influencing the experience of pain which can then be used to provide a rationale for the effective management of pain, taking into account the kinds of intervention that are available.

Armed with this information and the consequent picture it

provides of the pain experience the nurse or other health-care professional should be able to contribute much more effectively to the management of pain. This chapter considers therefore some of the administrative and organisational issues that can influence the delivery of good patient care in the management of pain.

Ethical issues

The management of pain must be seen as a priority of care (Copp 1985). There are many aspects of the ethics of care that can be seen as applying to pain. References in the nurses' Code of Professional Conduct (UKCC 1992a) to accountability, to levels of competence and keeping up to date impinge on the nurse's role in the management of pain as with any other aspect of care. In McCaffrey et al. (1994), arguments are made for the patient's right to the effective management of his or her pain. These include such issues as that the control of pain is a legitimate therapeutic goal; that it contributes significantly to the patient's physical and emotional well-being; that it ranks high in the lists of priorities in patient care; and that it can be patient controlled if the patient is communicative and the method safe. Issues of being informed and of patient choice are also considered.

There are a variety of principles that can be applied to guide our behaviour and our thinking in relation to ourselves and others. The subject of ethics is a huge one and one which has its own literature. Nevertheless four such principles have been suggested by Thompson et al. (1994) and variations on the same themes are offered in other texts which have been written especially for nurses or which are applicable to nursing situations, such as Beauchamp and Childress (1989) and Chadwick and Tadd (1992).

The four principles proposed in Thompson et al. (1994) are protective beneficence; justice or the respect for persons; justice and equity; and personal rights and autonomy. The first involves a caring ethic relating to an individualistic helping role, the protection of the weak and the role of advocacy. The second is concerned with reciprocal rights and responsibility, often seen in terms of contracts, formal or informal. A shared and agreed care plan could be seen as an example of such a contract, and recognition of what the nurse agrees to do and not to do and what the patient agrees to do and not to do. Issues of personal accountability and responsibility are dealt with under this principle. The third principle is that of public accountability and equity – as a member of a profession or of a particular community one must ensure that one treats or deals with others on an equal basis, and that one is so treated oneself. Finally the fourth principle covers the right of individuals to the exercise of personal autonomy, the right to participation and to the pursuit of individual happiness and fulfilment.

Professionals involved in the management of pain have to take each of these principles into consideration, as they must in any other professional area. Carr and Thomas (1997) develop a model of care for pain control based on those of Griepp (1992) and Ferrell *et al.* (1991). From this a strategy for decision making around a pain problem can be prepared, factors influencing the management of pain can be identified and dealt with, and the plan of care can be put into action. Perhaps the main point from this is that there is rarely a standard routine approach to any particular pain problem. Each situation must be seen as requiring an individual plan of care. This is particularly important in transcultural nursing, as discussed in Chapter 6 above. The importance of empathy and interpersonal skills to achieve such an individualised assessment and plan of care in the management of pain has been discussed by Davis (1990).

The nursing process

The well-established approach to the delivery of nursing care known as the nursing process is an obvious model for the management of pain (e.g. Roper *et al.* 1990). The stages or phases of assessment, planning, intervention and evaluation can be seen as reflecting the issues considered in the various chapters above. Chapter 9 dealt in detail with the ways in which pain can be assessed in a variety of pain situations. Without adequate assessment there cannot be adequate pain management. As with any aspect of care, the assessment determines the nature of problems and the kinds of interventions that might be applied.

This approach is also often called a problem-solving approach (Mayers 1978; Hunt and Marks-Maran 1986) as once the assessment has been made the problems identified must then be dealt with. This can involve consideration of a range of alternative interventions and consultation with other health-care professionals, and if possible the patient.

Assessment

Factors influencing the quality of the assessment include the nurse's level of knowledge and skill (e.g. Watt-Watson 1987; Dalton 1989; Fothergill-Bourbonnais and Wilson-Barnett 1992; Closs 1996), although there are differences between nurses working in different settings. For example, hospice workers had a higher level of knowledge than nurses in ITU (Fothergill-Bourbonnais and Wilson-Barnett 1992). There has also been noted a failure to use assessment tools or instruments to quantify the pain or to gain qualitative information (Hollingworth 1995). Camp-Sorrell and O'Sullivan (1987) have noted the poor quality of documentation of pain (also O'Connor 1995a, b), and similar reports have continued to appear regarding the documentation of the nursing process in general (Davis *et al.* 1994). With the elderly it has been found that there can be difficulties with the VAS or numerical scales; the six-point verbal scale seems to be more effective (Walker *et al.* 1990).

Nurses tend to under-estimate patients' pain (Seers 1987), and at an organisational level, poor policy decisions and inter-professional communication have been noted with reference to pain management (Evans 1992). Meurier *et al.* (1998) have identified the following factors as causing omissions in assessments: the patient's condition; work overload; lack of time; poor assessment documentation; not realising that the assessment had not been carried out; and different nurses being involved. Attitudes can be very influential, and Nash *et al.* (1993) found that intention to conduct pain assessment was predicted by attitude, subjective norms and perceived control. This latter seemed to have a particularly important independent effect. At an individual level there is evidence that social and cultural factors can influence nurses' attitudes and practice regarding pain (Davitz and Davitz 1981). There are of course many social and cultural factors affecting the pain experience of patients, and these can also influence the behaviour and thinking of the nurse or other health-care professional (see Chapter 6).

There are also misconceptions which play a part in the quality of assessment, and these have been well reviewed by McCaffrey *et al.* (1994). They include misconceptions about the veracity of the patient's report of pain (they may be lying to gain attention or some other gain), it is all in the mind anyway, or, if there are no physical signs, then there cannot be any pain. Other misconceptions include the omnipotence of the professional team regarding all pain issues and the belief that there are standard pains and standard remedies. It is of course vitally important that the person assessing pain must take into account the individual patient's responses to what they say is a pain experience as well as their own knowledge of the various factors that can influence that experience. The patient has a right to be heard and a right to be believed.

Planning

In many situations it is the nurse or the nursing team that is largely responsible for the assessment of pain and the application of most of the interventions. The multi-professional team is involved in the initial establishment of the assessment strategy but mainly in the planning stage, as the nature of the particular pain problems are identified and the most relevant interventions are determined, and prescribed.

The nature of the assessment will to a large extent determine the kind of planning that will take place. If as wide a range of aspects of the pain experience have been assessed as possible, then there will be a wide range of information available to consider in the planning process. In this way an account can be taken of the individual needs of the patient and a suitably individual programme of care identified. It is most important that the planning process is multi-disciplinary and that nurses in particular are involved. It can be argued that the nurse will bring a more holistic approach and also perhaps have direct experience of the patient.

Interventions

It is mainly nurses who are involved in the delivery of care in the management of pain. With respect to the actual application of interventions, some of the issues have been considered in the various chapters reviewing them. For example, with pharmacological interventions we have reviewed issues concerning fears of addiction, tolerance and dependence (see Chapter 7). With pharmacological interventions however it is important also that nurses are up to date with their knowledge of the actual drugs and also with the legislation covering their storage, prescription and administration.

The Misuse of Drugs Act 1971 and the Medicines Act 1968 (see Trounce 1997) and their respective Regulations cover the supply and use of drugs. The Misuse of Drugs Act covers drugs of addiction or controlled drugs, and various Schedules apply to some important analgesic preparations, such as Schedule 2 which means that drugs covered, such as morphine, must be under full control, under lock and key and with a register. Certain drugs can now be legally prescribed by nurses with special training for use in community settings, and midwives can carry and use pethidine as part of their practice (see Trounce 1997 for a discussion of these issues). There are also Standards for the Administration of Medicines for nurses (UKCC 1992b) with which all those involved in the management and administration of medicines should be familiar.

McCaffrey et al. (1994) argue for an active role for the nurse regarding interventions in general and pharmacological ones in particular. Generally it is the nurse who is involved in the preparation and delivery of an intervention unless it concerns intrathecal administration or technical equipment such as some PCA machines or physical therapies. The medical staff will be involved in assessment and the decision-making process about the nature of the problem and the intervention to be applied, although there is increasingly a multi-professional management of this aspect. It is important, argue McCaffrey et al. (1994), that the nurse is aware of this responsible, active and accountable role. It is the nurse's responsibility to maintain and up-date her or his level of competency and knowledge (UKCC 1992a).

Evaluation

In many ways this is the most important aspect of the nursing process. Yet it is all too frequently the area where the system breaks down (Davis et al. 1994). However, it is most important with respect to the management of pain (O'Connor 1995a, b). The cyclical nature of the nursing process would seem to be particularly suited to the regular monitoring of the outcomes of interventions for pain. Part of the planning process should include the determination of suitable outcomes that can be measured to demonstrate the effectiveness or otherwise of the intervention. In the acute pain setting it is important to get as good a result as possible as quickly as possible. Therefore each dose should be evaluated prior to the next being administered so that it may be changed or modified if necessary. It is through this process of titration that a satisfactory level of drug dose can be achieved. This is also important with chronic pain and with cancer pain, and the only way in which the analgesic ladder can be effectively implemented (World Health Organisation 1996). It is also important regarding the identification and treatment of side or toxic effects.

For the evaluation the nurse must be prepared to reassess the patient. The choice and use of the various instruments for this must be explored and considered carefully with respect to the frequency of evaluation and the time factors involved. It most probably will be that once a thorough, comprehensive assessment has been made at the beginning of treatment, then a relatively simple method of assessment of the intensity of the pain such as a VAS, numerical rating scale or six-point verbal scale may suffice for the evaluation. If other outcomes are being assessed then suitable indicators and instruments must be identified and utilised (see Chapter 9). The period between assessments of such outcomes may be relatively long term, if they involve interpersonal, social or work-related factors.

Other outcomes may involve negative aspects such as side effects or toxic effects of drug or other interventions. As we are aware that certain drugs and other forms of pain relief do generate side effects or can have toxic effects then we must be aware also of the need to monitor for these. Our plan of care should list all outcomes to be monitored, both those related to relief of pain and other positive outcomes and the likelihood of side effects or toxic effects. Suitable time-scales should be planned for their evaluation. Data about such common side effects as nausea and vomiting, constipation, or potentially serious ones such as depressed respiration could be being collected as part of the general care of the patients.

The results of the evaluation are then available to feed into the next planning phase. A review of the planned interventions in the light of evaluations can then be used to modify the interventions as necessary. This might mean an increase or decrease in a drug dose. Alternatively it may mean a different drug or the addition of another drug. It might mean the additional or alternative use of another from of treatment, such as a physical or psychological approach. Such planning review sessions should be shared by all members of the multi-professional team.

Special aspects of pain management

Acute pain services

These are relatively recent developments and largely came about in the UK as a result of the Report of the Royal Colleges (1990). Some experimental schemes began in the late 1980s (e.g. Wheatley *et al.* 1991). The structure usually consists of a multi-professional team, based around the consultant anaesthetist and involving one or more nurse specialists and perhaps a psychologist. In some situations it may be nurse led with the anaesthetist being consulted as necessary. Hunter (1993) has identified four main aims: the supervision of post-operative pain management; the application and advancement of new methods of analgesia; the support and education of the medical and nursing staff in new techniques; and finally the monitoring and improvement of the service. Evaluation of an acute pain service (APS) in West Yorkshire has demonstrated that there had been a significant impact on changing outcomes and improving quality of patient care (Mackintosh and Bowles 1997).

It is most important that there is good collaboration between the members of the different professional groups, and a clear definition of roles, particularly regarding leadership and responsibility for the various activities and decision making (Evans 1992). The overall model of care should be shared (Fagerhaugh and Strauss 1977) with a move towards more holistic approaches rather than a strict medical model.

The Acute Pain Team has, as a major role, the education and support of general nursing and other health-care professionals in the care of people in pain. Thus general day-to-day care of patients in pain should be part of their concern. However, if the pain problem becomes more complicated or the strategy of intervention is not effective then the team can become involved to plan a more effective approach. Some interventions may be the prerogative of the Acute Pain Team. The Team will have a special role in the auditing of the acute pain service; the amount of drugs used and with what effect; the introduction and evaluation of relatively new interventions such as PCA; the use of epidural analgesia; or the use of physical or psychological interventions. In order to facilitate this audit role it is most important that any documentation used is completed properly and made available for this central activity. This should include documented assessments as well as plans for and evaluations of care.

The Team should be involved at the pre-operative stage when the anaesthetist and perhaps the senior Pain Nurse makes an initial assessment at the beginning of the care plan. Generally the emphasis of assessment in the acute situation concerns the sensory-discriminatory aspects, the site, severity and nature of the pain. There might also be an interest in anxiety associated with the situation, such as pre-operatively or regarding trauma. Data should be collected as comprehensively as possible about these two aspects. There is a major role here regarding information giving in order to relieve as much anxiety as possible and to prepare the patient to cope more effectively as possible post-operatively (Hayward 1975; Davis 1984a; Johnson and Vogele 1993). Patient teaching in general is an important role for nurses in pain management (Wilson-Barnett 1997). This is then picked up and developed immediately post-operatively. It may involve also staff in intensive care. Once on the ward then the Team should make regular rounds to monitor the management of the patient's pain. The acute pain may be associated with a medical emergency rather than a surgical or trauma situation. However, the same principles should apply.

Chronic pain clinics

A similar service has been developed for chronic pain patients as that described above for the acute pain patient. There is however a longer history behind this kind of service. Bonica described the establishment of a chronic pain service as long ago as 1974. The clinic generally comprises a team of specialists including anaesthetists, nurses and psychologists. Diamond and Coniam (1991) argue that the chronic pain clinic (CPC) is a Pain Management Service, whereby not only is there an attempt to relieve the pain but also to deal with the suffering and disability (the cognitive and social aspects) as well. Much of the work of the CPC involves the use of psychological interventions, and some physical ones, although the use of pharmacological interventions is a mainstay. However, the use of pharmacological interventions in the long-term situation can be problematic and therefore the adjunctive use of psychological and physical interventions can be most valuable (see previous chapters on the various interventions).

The main objectives of pain-management programmes run in CPCs are to increase self-perceived control over pain; to increase self-perceived independence; to increase levels of physical and social activity; and to reduce levels of emotional distress (Diamond and Coniam 1991). Melzack and Wall (1996) identify three advantages to CPCs: the first is educational where in a multi-professional team professionals learn from each other; the second is the potential for the development of new therapies, particularly psychological and physical ones; and the third is the potential for the accumulation of data regarding the effectiveness of treatment and of the service.

As with the acute pain service, the essence of the CPC is the multi-disciplinary team. However, similarly there is a key role for the nurse in such a team, as the kinds of intervention for which they can be responsible can provide much comfort and relief to the patient. The process with a new patient referred to the clinic should involve an initial interview with the anaesthetist and the nurse to identify the nature of the pain problem. Aspects to be covered will include the site, severity and nature of the pain and also the length of time it has been present. These are the sensory-discriminatory aspects. However, there is always as much concern with the emotional-motivational, cognitive-evaluative and social-cultural aspects. The assessment is holistic and the range of interventions that might be used for the plan of care will similarly be holistic, embracing pharmacological, psychological and physical approaches, such as those described in Chapters 7 and 8 above (Diamond and Coniam 1991). Generally the CPC deals with chronic non-malignant pain. However, cancer pain is a major part of chronic pain, and special services, such as hospices and palliative care services, have been established to help people in that situation.

Patient teaching

The nurse, in both acute and chronic pain settings, can have a very important part to play regarding information giving and patient education. Communication and interpersonal aspects of care have long been advocated as being a most valuable part of the nursing role (e.g. Davis 1981). Evidence has accrued over the last twenty-five years demonstrating in particular the therapeutic role that can be undertaken by nurses in for example pre-operative information giving (e.g. Hayward 1975; Boore 1978; Davis 1984a in the UK; and Johnson and Vogele 1993 in the USA). Patient education is also an important aspect of chronic pain management. It plays a significant part, in particular, with regard to the work of CPCs (see Melzack and Wall 1996).

Hospices and palliative pain services

Cancer pain is seen as being different from non-malignant pain (Sofaer 1998). There are aspects of death and dying always at the back of the perception of the pain, as well as its progressive nature. One of the first hospice services was St Christopher's in London (Saunders 1978, 1994). Hospices are generally charitable organisations outside the health service but obviously complementary to it. They specialise in the care of people in pain from cancer and those who are dying. They tend to offer a flexible service, which offers continuing care or respite care. Many hospices and palliative care services are organised under the auspices of national charities such as Marie Curie Cancer Care and Macmillan Cancer Relief. Some palliative services are hospital based too, such as that developed by Ajemian and Mount (1980).

Some argue that hospice and palliative care is not only terminal care (Fisher 1991). Four types of care offered by hospices can be identified (Pearce 1993).These are pain and symptom control; rehabilitation; respite care; and continuing or terminal care. The length of terminal care can vary from a few weeks to a few years (McCusker 1983). One of the problems is in the definition of a health problem as becoming 'terminal' (Davis *et al.* 1996). Many professionals, particularly doctors, find it difficult to admit that a particular situation offers no more hope and the patient is in a 'dying trajectory'. Perhaps this reflects their general 'cure' orientation, as opposed to the 'care' orientation of other professionals. However, many doctors do have a 'care' orientation and are more willing to make an earlier diagnosis of a terminal state. Care provided by hospice and palliative services can vastly improve the quality of life in the final period (Doyle 1986). A wide range of treatments are always available for the management of pain as well as the coming to terms with approaching death, particularly involving psychiatric and psycho-social aspects (Cherny and Portenoy 1994; Breitbart *et al.* 1994).

There are still many problems associated with understanding the nature of cancer and cancer care, including the management of pain (McCaffrey *et al.* 1994; Richardson 1997). These can include knowledge of doctors and nurses; the knowledge of patients and their families; the time available for the care process; and conflicts between doctors and nurses about under- or over-medication. Some of these involve patient teaching and professional education. These have been identified as being responsibilities and functions of APSs and CPCs and they are also important for hospice and palliative care services. Indeed both Marie Curie Cancer Care and Macmillan Cancer Relief employ education staff, or staff with an education role, as part of their support systems. The author has been and currently is actively involved in negotiating, along with medical colleagues, with both these organisations for such hospice and university-based appointments. Patient teaching and professional education are considered in more detail below.

Pain in children and infants

Evidence has been referred to above about poor management of pain in children and infants (Schechter *et al.* 1986; P. A. McGrath 1990; Cummings *et al.* 1996), and some aspects of the use of pharmacological preparations, psychological and physical treatments have been considered, as well as the assessment of pain in children. The sensory-discriminative, the emotional and motivational, the cognitive-evaluative, and the social aspects of the pain experience have also been referred to in the various chapters dealing with those issues. In this section these points will be brought together and summarised to aid the general picture of pain in children and infants.

The evidence seems to be convincing that very young children, even neonates, can experience something that adults would call pain (e.g. Anand and Hickey 1987; McGrath and Unruh 1994). There is some evidence that to a certain extent they may be more sensitive to pain than adults (Fowler-Kerry and Lander 1987). The nociceptive processes deliver pain stimuli to the central nervous system, where, as the cognitive abilities of the infant develop, the pain becomes more and more meaningful with increasing age. Much of this meaning is learned from adults through role modelling (Bandura 1977). However, young children may have difficulty in expressing the pain in a way that is easy for adults to understand. Great skill is needed to assess pain in young children and a variety of instruments and techniques have been developed although there is room for more research. The role of parents is vitally important in assessing pain and in the administration of interventions.

There is a wide variety of interventions to help even the neonate in pain and it is important that the potential is realised when planning care (see Chapters 8 and 9). There are safe pharmacological preparations and some psychological and physical interventions that should meet most needs. The role of the nurse as advocate for the child is very important to combat any misconceptions that might continue to exist and interfere with the management of pain (Akinsanya 1985).

McCaffrey *et al.* (1994) have identified some of these misconceptions. One of these is that denial of pain means the child does not feel any pain. There is often such a fear of the intervention (particularly needles) that pain will be denied to avoid that. Another misconception is that if a child can be distracted or get to sleep then there cannot have been much pain. With distraction the pain is still there but the attention of the child (as with an adult) can be distracted for a relatively short period. Similarly children do not tolerate pain better than adults. Pharmacological preparations are no more dangerous with children and infants than with adults. Side effects and toxic effects can be avoided or treated (Lynn and Slattery 1987), and addiction is so rare as not to be a problem (Schechter *et al.* 1988). Some people think that as pain is not life threatening, and the child will not remember the incident anyway, then there is no need to provide analgesia. The reverse is all too true. Children do remember pain and the shock reaction to untreated acute or chronic pain can be very debilitating and make worse any other threat to life (Beaver 1987).

Nurses have a great potential in the care of pain in children and infants. Because of the relationships that they can build with children and their parents there is much information that they can receive from both that can help in the determination of the nature of the pain and possible interventions and plans of care. However, this close involvement, particularly if for long periods of time, can lead to emotional stress in those nurses which can have deleterious effects on their health and ability to function properly (Nagy 1998).

The role of parents in the management of children in general has been advocated by Palmer (1993) and Darbyshire (1993) although the latter also notes some of the problems. Abu-Saad and Hamers (1997) also note the importance of the information that may be gained from parents. There is also the potential for much patient and parent teaching as a result of that relationship. This includes the correction of misconceptions on the part of children and their parents as well as giving information about the nature of pain and the pro's and con's of the various interventions. Parents can also be supported and encouraged to contribute to the care by participating with some of the interventions.

The elderly

There is an increasing tendency to treat the elderly (however defined) as a different group much as children and infants have been. However, there is no evidence that they lose their sensitivity to pain, that they are more susceptible to respiratory depression or that they are less trustworthy regarding reports of pain (e.g. Closs 1996). There is perhaps a tendency to report less pain, but this is more likely to be because they have developed coping strategies of their own (e.g. Walker *et al.* 1990; Corran *et al.* 1994). They can be very vulnerable to psychological and social factors (Roy 1992). In an important study of the experience of pain in the elderly, Walker *et al.* (1989, 1990) identified a range of factors that influence pain in this group. These included the amount of information they feel they had received; the development of personal strategies for coping; the ability to keep occupied; having regrets; having non-pain-related problems; and loneliness. This study also produced a model for the management of pain in the elderly which could act as a model for any patient in chronic pain.

Growing old brings with it many degenerative changes which can cause pain, particularly joint pains. Many elderly people also become depressed. This may also be associated with pain. The evidence seems to be however that the pain causes the depression rather than vice versa (e.g. Ahles *et al.* 1987). However, depression can exacerbate the experience of pain and interfere with motivation and coping, which is a different thing (see Chapter 4). In a review article on the management of pain in the elderly, Gagliese and Melzack (1997) identify three main aspects that warrant attention. These are inappropriate assessment strategies; concerns about adverse effects of pharmacological preparations; and misconceptions about pain in the elderly. With respect to treatments, the evidence seems to suggest that the elderly would benefit from a multi-modal approach and in particular from psychological treatment methods. With respect to the misconceptions, it seems that pain is as intense with the elderly as with other age groups. Pain is not a normal part of ageing and always warrants treatment.

In many instances again, it is the nurse who is most involved with the elderly person in pain, particularly in the community. The quality of the relationship it is possible to establish in these circumstances provides an excellent opportunity to gain as much information as possible from the person in pain and to give as much information as possible or as is required. In many ways the elderly will have a life-time of experience to help them but this same experience may also have a negative influence. The nurse can offer supportive or correc-tive input as necessary.

The full range of interventions is available for the elderly including pharmacology and particularly the psycho-social strategies. There is no increased danger from opioids with the elderly (Portenoy and Foley 1986). Lack of information and loneliness can be dealt with through psycho-social interventions and many physical therapies have been used with success in support of the strategies developed by the elderly people themselves. Working with the patient and supporting their own approach to their pain can be very effective (Walker *et al.* 1990). As with all people in pain, it is essentially their pain. The experience of it and its meaning is theirs and we can only come in from the outside to help them through the experience. We can add information and interventions and provide support and together provide a more effective antidote to this most frightening and dreaded phenomenon.

Audit

The problems identified above in the management of pain, and the amount of evidence demonstrating relatively poor quality of care in many cases, suggest that the introduction of regular audit of pain management might help to prevent these. The Association of Anaesthetists of Great Britain and Ireland together with the Pain Society argue that this should be part of the annual business plan (1997). Such audits should address effectiveness, efficiency and quality. Justins (1998) has reported on the GMC's appointment of the Pain and Palliative Medicine Liaison Group in an attempt to improve practice in pain management. It is important that nurses should be looking to audit their part in the management of pain, particularly those provided by APSs and CPCs. Publication of lessons learnt and suggestions for the improvement of services could be usefully shared with colleagues.

Conclusion

This chapter has emphasised the importance of an ethical base to practice. It is most important that rights and responsibilities are clearly understood by the professionals providing a pain service. It is also important that we help the person in pain, and their family if necessary, to appreciate these aspects. Many misconceptions exist about pain, particularly regarding children and the elderly, but also with the adult and it is most important that accurate information is available for nurses and other health-care professionals as well as for patients.

The special needs of particular groups have been identified and points raised to illustrate how misconceptions can be corrected and particular needs be catered for. These have included children and the very young infant and neonate, as well as the elderly, at the other end of the life continuum. The important point is that from viable birth to death we can and do experience pain and the needs of the individual in pain are no less at any particular point in the life trajectory. There are however special aspects to the needs of individuals with different kinds of pain and at different stages of growth, development and when growing old. The individualised approach to care that is nowadays advocated for the management of pain, based on the realisation that pain is very much an individual phenomenological experience, is the only way that these special needs can be met.

In developing a programme of care it is imperative that it is a structured and research-based approach. The nursing process, as an example of an individualised, problem-solving approach, has been offered, and the various stages or phases illustrated to demonstrate how it could be utilised. Although this approach is recommended for the general management of pain, it is also the approach recommended when special pain services are established. It has been realised that the management of pain is now a clinical speciality. Many nurses are now employed as clinical nurse specialists in this area managing or collaborating in pain services, either in the acute setting, with the management of chronic pain, or in hospice or palliative care.

A major advantage of a managed pain service, such as an APS or a CPC, is the collection of data about the service so that regular monitoring and auditing of the quality of care can be undertaken. Documentation of the number of cases; the amount of pain; the use of drugs and other physical and psychological interventions; the level and nature of outcome achieved is essential. It is only if we have this kind of regular information that we will be able to improve the quality of care. In this way we can then ensure that the most effective interventions are used to meet the degree and kind of pain experienced by each of the people who come into our care.

Chapter 11

Conclusion

The future – research and education

This volume so far has described the current state of our understanding of the pain experience and of the interventions and strategies available for its management and the care of people in pain. It is hoped that the picture given of the kind of experiences people in pain have, covering the sensory-discriminative, the emotional and motivational, the cognitive-evaluative, and the socio-cultural, will facilitate a better rationale for practice. Professionals, particularly nurses, from such a knowledge base as this, should then be able to develop and implement care plans for any individual, dealing with that person's particular experience.

However, situations change, new insights or problems emerge from practice or from research, and there is a continuing need to continue our search for knowledge and for us to be continually updating ourselves as professionals in the light of the developing knowledge base. In this last chapter of the book we shall consider the issues of generating or developing new knowledge through research and of preparing practitioners in the light of the insights given in the preceding chapters and of any new knowledge that might be gained. Finally an overview of the whole book will be given to demonstrate the value of the 'inside story' in caring for people in pain

Research

There are three main areas for future research: the patient's experience across the four dimensions discussed above; the various kinds of interventions; and the management of pain. Each of these areas is of course multi-factorial and involves a wide variety of experts and professionals. What follows is a brief attempt to indicate avenues for future research in each of these three.

At the sensory-discriminatory level of the experience there is increasing activity as more and more sophisticated techniques are developed. The gate control model, increasingly supported, is however being shown not to be the relatively simplistic mechanism proposed in 1965 by Melzack and Wall. They themselves have contributed to the understanding of the increasingly complicated system that seems to be operating, at the periphery, in the dorsal horn, in the various levels of the ascending and descending spinal tracts, the midbrain areas and the cortex (Melzack and Wall 1996). Recent conference proceedings demonstrate the high level of activity in all of these areas (Jensen *et al.* 1997). Some of these findings have been incorporated into this volume, as have more recent findings from journals and research reports.

A particularly difficult area to study is that of the emotional, motivational and behavioural aspects of the pain experience. This is perhaps made more difficult because of the interaction between physiological, biochemical and cognitive processes. The assessment of pain in neonates and young infants is a particularly important area (Grunau *et al.* 1994). Similarly the cognitive and social meanings of the pain experience are a compound of cortical neuronal activity and the learning, memory, problem solving and thinking processes at a more abstract level. Recent developments in the visualisation of neuronal activity in relation to these abstract processes, utilising PET scans (Jones 1997; Treede *et al.* 1999), could be opening the door to a new kind of insight into the pain experience. This would achieve the integration of the four levels of experience that currently exist largely as separate entities.

Research into the various interventions progresses very well regarding the development of new analgesics or new refined versions of the old ones. The problem of side effects is an area for future research. As we get more powerful analgesics for example we have to find more powerful drugs or techniques to combat the side effects which make treatment problematic. Following an historical and scientific review of cannabis for the treatment of pain, in particular migraine, Russo (1998) argues for controlled clinical trials of the drug in the management of acute migraine. Development of versions of the analgesics that are particularly suitable for young children and infants is also an area of need, and Hermann *et al.* (1995) argue for more comparisons between pharmacological and behavioural interventions. There are also many aspects of the psychology of pain that warrant further research, particularly those aspects associated with attempts to measure quality of life and the effect of pain, as well as the cognitive-evaluative aspects (Skevington 1995).

One of the major problems with physical and psychological treatments has been the difficulty in generating suitable research designs so that a clear cause-and-effect link can be established. A particular issue here is perhaps the failure to ask the most relevant research question or, more particularly, to define the most apt outcome to be measured. Many of the physical and psychological interventions do not have a great effect on the intensity of pain (Broome *et al.* 1989; Sindhu 1996; Seers and Carroll 1998; Carroll and Seers 1998). However, these interventions do seem to have potential benefit in terms of more emotional, motivational or cognitive-evaluative outcomes, and could be used in a variety of settings including accident and emergency departments (Herbert 1998). There is perhaps too narrow a focus on pain intensity as the most desired outcome of research. Also there is perhaps too much dependence on the 'gold standard' of the randomised controlled trial as the preferred design. Lewith and Aldridge (1993) have reviewed a variety of research strategies that could offer alternatives and yet provide evidence of clinical effectiveness that is acceptable, with particular reference to the complementary therapies. They include the use of quasi-experimental designs, case studies and action research designs, as well as discussing the importance of control and bias. More recently Rolfe (1998) has argued for single-case studies, action research and reflective case studies.

Finally it is perhaps most important that research activity is increasingly multi-professional and multi-disciplinary. The problems within each of the four dimensions of the pain experience as well as their integration, and the problems relating to the various interventions, are more likely to be addressed with input from nurses and physiotherapists for example as well as from psychologists and socio-economists.

Education

The problem

Evidence has already been given of the relatively poor quality of pain management (e.g. Donovan *et al.* 1987; The Royal Colleges

1990; Alleyne and Thomas 1994). To a large extent this seems to be linked to poor levels of knowledge by nurses (Sofaer 1984; Watt-Watson 1987; Dalton 1989; Fothergill-Bourbonnais and Wilson-Barnett 1992; McCaffrey *et al.* 1994). These studies have involved surveys of practising nurses in a variety of settings including hospices and ITU. Generally nurses feel poorly prepared and fail to answer questions of knowledge correctly. What is particularly upsetting with these findings is the failure to demonstrate improvement over the years.

There is also evidence of poor practice, for example a failure to use well-established and evaluated tools (Walker *et al.* 1990); poor assessment (K. Seers 1987); poor documentation of information (Camp-Sorrell and O'Sullivan 1991; O'Connor 1995a, b; Davis *et al.* 1994); and under-administration of analgesics, particularly with children (e.g. Beyer and Byers 1985). The development of educational programmes based on these insights and the knowledge of the patients' experience and interventions considered in the previous chapters, it is hoped, should help to improve matters.

In a small-scale study Sofaer (1984) did demonstrate an improvement in achievement of pain relief following the introduction of an educational programme, as did Davis with a staff-initiated programme (1988a). He demonstrated changes in attitude through the development of an assessment tool. Gadish *et al.* (1988) and Hamers *et al.* (1994) also found that a higher level of education led to an increased likelihood of administration of higher doses of opioids. However, Heaven and Maguire (1996) found that improvements of assessment procedures were not necessarily enough to improve the quality of pain relief. Attitudes and beliefs are also important, as is an increased sensitivity to the patient's experience of pain. De Rond *et al.* (1999), in The Netherlands, developed an educational programme regarding guidelines for the assessment of pain using a numeric rating scale on a daily basis. Nurse compliance was high and patients were positive about the daily assessment regime using this instrument.

What to teach

There is evidence that there is relatively poor coverage of pain issues in nursing curricula (Davis and Seers 1991; Franke *et al.* 1996). As well as covering information about the four dimensions of the pain experience, and the various kinds of interventions, education must also deal with attitudes and feelings (Sofaer 1998). This should tackle some of the many misconceptions about the pain experience and strategies for management. There have been attempts to generate model curricula to guide the development of local courses for those involved in the management of pain. One of the most detailed is that published by the International Association for the Study of Pain (IASP) (Fields 1995). This is a research-based curriculum covering all aspects of the pain experience, interventions and detailed consideration of special pain situations. The IASP have also published a pain curriculum for basic nurse education. Berde (1993) and both Davis and Seers (1991) and Seers and Davis (1993) have discussed this aspect. Again they emphasise the importance of attitudes to support the application of knowledge in practice.

An important aspect however is the application of knowledge into practice. Skills are as important as the knowledge base, as is the question of level. All practitioners should have some input on the management of pain in their pre-registration programmes. However, there is much need for advanced studies to enable the developing practitioners to enhance the level of their practice as they perhaps take on more specialist roles. King (1997) has identified four levels of practice, based on the work of Benner (1984) and others. These are beginner, competent practitioner, proficient practitioner and expert. In her relatively small-scale study King (1997) showed how the intensive care nurses moved from dependence, a learner role, task orientation and more rigid, rule-following practice, towards more independence and autonomy, more of a teaching role, a more patient centred, holistic and flexible approach. There are examples of post-registration diploma and master's-level programmes now operating to enable practitioners to develop increasing levels of knowledge and skills to be able to offer increasingly advanced and insightful programmes of care. Some of these are also multi-professional.

In an attempt to enhance the role of the nurse and to develop a more holistic approach many nurses are showing an interest in training in complementary therapies. This could be of particular value with some of the specialist situations (Closs 1996). Another important aspect of skills training is that of interpersonal and communications skills. The educational role of the nurse particularly with regard to patient teaching is most important (Wilson-Barnett 1997), as has been shown with regard to the value of pre-operative information giving for example (Johnson and Vogele 1993). With particular reference to the transcultural situation, communication is vitally important and particularly the role of empathy (Davis 1990). Empathy is important with all patients of course. Recent reviews of the value of complementary therapies seem to indicate that it is information giving, and the time taken to talk to patients, a hallmark of these approaches, that is the effective factor (as noted following systematic reviews by Broome *et al.* (1989) and Sindhu (1996)). More focused research as indicated above could help to clarify this.

How to teach

As pain management is increasingly multi-professional and team based it would seem to make sense to educate the members of the team together. Inter-professional education in the area of health-care studies is now a developing force, and the area of pain management could be a leader. As well as being inter-professional the educational strategy should not only be concerned with the acquisition of facts but the development of decision-making skills and attitudes.

A problem-based approach to education is demonstrating advantages over the more traditional didactic approach (Andrews and Jones 1996). By working together in small groups of professionals perhaps from the same team, the students could be presented with real-life scenarios and asked to derive, as a team, a strategy for care that meets the holistic needs of the particular client. Discussions of roles as well as assessment and planning of interventions should occur. Arguments based on research should accompany all final plans. This kind of approach is particularly suitable for part-time or distance-learning programmes where the students may bring from their practice problems to be considered as part of the course.

Professional organisations

Many practitioners work in relative isolation or as members of small teams. It is important that staff keep in touch with the general subject, and not only through reading journals. Membership of professional organisations can help by being involved with a larger perhaps specialist, uni- or multi-professional group, at both the national and international level. For nurses there is the RCN Pain Forum and the Acute Pain Network. The Pain Society in the UK is a multi-professional group that organises major international annual conferences. Nurses are becoming increasingly influential as their membership grows. The Pain Society is affiliated to the IASP and as such participates in the international conferences of that organisation. Again nurses are participating increasingly in the IASP and presenting papers and posters at its conferences. Addresses of these organisations are given in the Appendix (p. 209).

Conclusion

Thus we come to the end of this book. The 'inside story' has been told and used as a basis for the consideration of methods of treatment, assessment and administration of interventions to help people in pain. There is now much evidence available about the different aspects of this 'inside story', much more than it has been possible to reference in the volume. This evidence indicates that except for some very special situations, most people in pain should be able to obtain relief within a relatively short time and for the necessary length of time.

Problems have been identified with the care of people in pain, and a variety of factors exposed. The bottom line however seems to be that there is the knowledge but the skills and attitudes need attention. Weaknesses in the system have been mentioned and these form the basis of proposals for developments in education, practice and, of course, further research.

The story began with the sensory-discriminative aspects of the pain experience, where we followed the track of the stimulus through the nervous system to the central parts of the brain where awareness becomes involved and there are the emotional and motivational aspects to the experience. There is a close physiological relationship between the sensory-discriminative and emotional-motivational aspects, with the same structures and processes being involved with both. This gives the pain experience a much more holistic aspect.

However, when we get to the cognitive-evaluative aspects we have a third dimension that is also intricately linked with the previous two, as the meaning of the situation gives added information that influences both the emotional-motivational and sensory-discriminative aspects, and thus the nature of the pain that is experienced. This cognitive-evaluative aspect is linked also with the social-cultural aspects which add to the meaning of the situation and the ways in which the pain is expressed.

We thus have a four-dimensional 'inside story' of the pain experience from which to gain an individual picture for a particular individual sufferer. This then can provide the basis for the development of a care plan, following an assessment process that taps all of these dimensions. This assessment process will vary in different care situations and with respect to the available resources and personnel. However, the principles should be the same and attempts made to achieve as four-dimensional a picture as possible.

Taking note of the weakness identified in the literature, about lack of knowledge, poor assessment skills, under-medication and so on, and the proposals for educational and practice developments, it should be possible to develop and run effective pain services. There is evidence that there is good practice. This should be audited and shared with others, through the evaluation and publication of developments in practice.

A very good measure of the quality of health care is the quality of the management of pain. It is hoped that this volume will help in the preparation and development of staff involved in this work, and thus ensure that we not only are concerned with the pain, but care for the people in pain.

Appendix
Useful organisations

Acute Pain Network
c/o Debbie Hunter
Pain Sister
York District General Hospital
Wiggington Road
York YO31 8HE

International Association for the Study of Pain
IASP Secretary
909 NE 43rd Street, Suite 306
Seattle, WA 98105–6020

The Pain Society of Great Britain and Northern Ireland
9 Bedford Square
London WC1B 3RA

The Royal College of Nursing Pain Forum
20 Cavendish Square
London W1M 0AB

For standards and code of professional conduct:

The United Kingdom Central Council for Nursing, Midwifery and
  Health Visiting
23 Portland Place
London W1N 4JT

References

Abramson, L. J., Seligman, M. E. P. and Teasdale, J. D. (1978) 'Learned helplessness in humans: critique and reformulation', *Journal of Abnormal Psychology* 87. 49

Abramson, L. J., Metalsky, G. I. and Alloy, L. A. (1989) 'Hopelessness depression – a theory based subtype of depression', *Psychological Review* 96. 2. 358–372

Abu-Saad, H. (1984) 'Assessing children's responses to pain', *Pain* 19. 163–171

—— (1990) 'Toward the development of an instrument to assess pain in children', Dutch study in D. C. Tyler and E. J. Krane (eds) *Advances in Pain Research and Therapy: Paediatric Pain* (Raven Press, New York)

Abu-Saad, H. H. and Hamers, J. P. H. (1997) 'Decision-making and paediatric pain: a review', *Journal of Advanced Nursing* 26. 946–952

Affleck, G., Tennen, H., Pfeiffer, C. and Fifield, J. (1987) 'Appraisals of control and predictability in adapting to chronic disease', *Journal of Personality and Social Psychology* 53. 273–279

Ahles, T. A., Yunus, M. B. and Masi, A. T. (1987) 'Is chronic pain a variant of depressive disease? The case of primary fibromyalgia syndrome', *Pain* 29. 105–111

Ajemian, I. and Mount, B. M. (eds) (1980) *The RVH on Palliative/Hospice Care* (Arno Press, New York)

Akinsanya, C. Y. (1985) 'The use of knowledge in the management of pain: the nurse's role', *Nurse Education Today* 5. 41–46

Alderfer, C. P. (1989) 'Theories reflecting my personal experience and life development', *Journal of Applied Behavioural Science* 25. 351–365

Alleyne, J. and Thomas, V. J. (1994) 'The management of sickle cell crisis pain as experienced by patients and carers', *Journal of Advanced Nursing* 19. 725–732

Anand, K. J. S., Brown, M. J. and Causson, R. C. (1985) 'Can the human neonate mount an endocrine/metabolic response to surgery?', *Journal of Pediatric Surgery* 20. 41–48

Anand, K. J. S. and Hickey, P. R. (1987) 'Pain and its effects in the human neonate and fetus', *New England Journal of Medicine* 317. 1,321–1,329

Anderson, A. D. and Pennebaker, J. W. (1980) 'Pain and pleasure: an alternative interpretation for identical stimulation', *European Journal of Social Psychology* 10. 2. 207–212

Anderson, J. R. (1983) *The Architecture of Cognition* (Harvard University Press, Cambridge MA)

Andrews, M. and Jones, P. R. (1996) 'Problem-based learning in an undergraduate nursing programme: a case study', *Journal of Advanced Nursing* 23. 2. 357–365

Aradine, C. R., Beyer, J. E. and Tompkins, J. M. (1987) 'Children's pain perception before and after analgesia: a study of instrument construct validity and related issues', *Journal of Pediatric Nursing* 3. 11–23

Armstrong, D. (1983) 'The fabrication of nurse/patient relationships', *Social Science and Medicine* 17. 457–460

Association of Anaesthetists of Great Britain and Ireland and The Pain Society (1997) *Provision of Pain Services* (Association of Anaesthetists, London)

Baird, P. (1934) 'On emotional expression after decortication with some remarks on certain theoretical views', *Psychological Review* 41. 309–328

Bandura, A. (1967) 'The role of modeling personality development', in C. Lavatelli and F. Stendler (eds) *Readings in Childhood and Development* (Harcourt Brace Jovanovich, New York)

—— (1971) 'Analysis of modeling processes', in A. Bandura (ed.) *Psychological Modeling* (Aldine Atherton, New York)

—— (1977) 'Self efficacy: toward a unifying theory of behavioural change', *Psychological Review* 84. 191–215

—— (1991) 'Social cognitive theory of self regulation', *Organisational Behaviour and Human Decision Processes* 50. 248–287

Baron, R. (1998) 'The influence of sympathetic nerve activity and catecholamines on primary afferent neurons', *IASP Newsletter* May/June

Baron, R. A. and Byrne, D. (1984) *Social Psychology: Understanding Human Interaction* 4th edn (Allyn and Bacon, Boston MA)

Bartlett, F. C. (1932) *Remembering* (Cambridge University Press, Cambridge)

Basbaum, A. I. and Fields, H. L. (1978) 'Endogenous pain control mechanisms: review and hypothesis', *Annals of Neurology* 4. 451–462

Bates, J. A. V. and Mathan, P. W. (1980) 'Transcutaneous electrical nerve stimulation for chronic pain', *Anaesthesia* 35. 817–822

Beail, N. (ed.) (1985) *Repertory Grid Technique and Personal Constructs. Applications in Clinical and Educational Settings* (Croom Helm, London)

Beauchamp, T. L. and Childress, J. F. (1989) *Principles of Biomedical Ethics* (Open University Press, Milton Keynes)

Beaver, P. K. (1987) 'Premature infants' response to touch and pain: can nurses make a difference?', *Neonatal Network* 6. 13–17

Beck, A. T. (1976) *Cognitive Therapy and Emotional Disorders* (International Universities Press, New York)

Beck, A. T., Rush, A. J., Shaw, B. F. and Emery, G. (1979) *Cognitive Therapy of Depression* (Guilford, New York)

Beck, A. T., Emery, G. and Greenberg, R. (1985) *Anxiety Disorders and Phobias: A Cognitive Perspective* (Basic Books, New York)

Beck, A. T., Steer, R. A. and Garbin, M. G. (1988) 'Psychometric properties of the Beck Depression Inventory: twenty-five years of evaluation', *Clinical Psychology Review* 8. 77–100

Becker, N., Bondegaard Thomsen, A., Olsen, A. K., Sjogren, P. and Erikson, J. (1997) 'Pain epidemiology and health related quality of life in chronic non-malignant pain patients referred to a Danish multidisciplinary pain center', *Pain* 73. 393–400

Becker, N., Hojsted, J., Sjogren, P. and Erikson, J. (1998) 'Sociodemographic predictors of treatment outcome in chronic non-malignant pain patients. Do patients receiving or applying for Disability Pension benefit from multidisciplinary pain treatment?', *Pain* 77. 279–287

Beecher, H. K. (1959) *Measurement of Subjective Responses* (Oxford University Press, New York)

Benner, P. (1984) *From Novice to Expert: Excellence and Power in Clinical Nursing Practice* (Addison-Wesley, Menlo Park CA)

—— (1985) 'Quality of Life: A phenomenological perspective on explanation, prediction and understanding in nursing science', *Advances in Nursing Science* 8. 1. 1–14

Benson, H. (1975) *The Relaxation Response* (William Morrow, New York)

Benson, H., Kotch, J. B., Crassweller, K. D. and Greenwood, M. M. (1977) 'Historical and clinical considerations of the relaxation response', *American Scientist* 65. 441–445

Benson, H., Pomeranz, B. and Kutz, I. (1984) 'The relaxation response and pain', in P. D. Wall and R. Melzack (eds) *Textbook of Pain* 1st edn (Churchill Livingstone, Edinburgh)

Bentley, J. (1998) 'The science of pain: an update', in B. Sofaer *Pain: Principles Practice and Patients* (Stanley Thornes, Cheltenham)

Berde, C. B. (ed.) (1993) 'Pain curriculum for basic nurse education', *IASP Newsletter* Sept.–Oct. Technical Corner (International Association for the Study of Pain, Seattle)

Berde, C. B., Holzman, R. S., Sethna, N. F., Dickerson, R. B. and Brustowicz, R. M. (1988) 'A comparison of methadone and morphine for post-operative analgesia in children and adolescents', *Anesthesiology* 69

Berde, C. B., Lehn, B. N. and Yee, Y. D. (1993) 'Patient controlled analgesia in children and adolescents: a randomised prospective comparison with intramuscular morphine for postoperative analgesia', *Pediatrics* 118. 460–466

Beyer, J. (1984) *The Oucher: A User's Manual and Technical Report* (The Hospital Play Equipment Co., Evanston IL)

Beyer, J. E. and Byers, M. L. (1985) 'Knowledge of pediatric pain: the state of the art', *Children's Health Care* 13. 150–159

Beyer, J. E., McGrath, P. J. and Berde, C. (1990) 'Discordance between self report and behavioural pain measures in 3–7 year old children following surgery', *Journal of Pain and Symptom Management* 5. 350–356

Beyer, J. E., Deynes, M. J. and Villareu, A. M. (1992) 'The creation, validation and continuing development of the Oucher: a measure of pain intensity in children', *Journal of Pediatric Nursing. Nursing Care of Children and Families* 7. 5. 335–346

Bibace, R. and Walsh, M. E. (1980) 'Development of children's concept of illness', *Pediatrics* 66. 912–917

Bieri, D., Reeve, R. A. and Champion, G. D. (1990) 'The Faces Pain Scale for the self assessment of the severity of the pain experienced by children: development, initial validation and preliminary investigation for ratio scale properties', *Pain* 41. 139–150

Black, D. (1992) 'Ethical issues arising from measures of quality of life', in A. H. Hopkins (ed.) *Measures of the Quality of Life and the Uses to Which Such Measures May Be Put* (Royal College of Physicians, London)

Black, R. G. (1975) 'The chronic pain syndrome', *Surgical Clinics of America* 55. 999–1,011

Blaxter, M. and Paterson, E. (1982) *Mothers and Daughters: A Three-Generational Study of Health Attitudes and Behaviour* (Heinemann, London)

Bokan, J. A., Ries, R. K. and Katon, W. J. (1981) 'Tertiary gain and chronic pain', *Pain* 10. 331–335

Bolles, R. C. and Franslow, M. S. (1980) 'A perceptual/defensive/recuperative model of fear in pain', *Behaviour and Brain Sciences* 3. 291–323

Bond, S. (1978) 'Processes of communication with cancer patients', in J. Wilson Barnett (ed.) *Nursing Research: Ten Studies in Patient Care* (John Wiley and Sons, Chichester)

Bonica, J. J. (1974) 'Organisation and function of a pain clinic', in J. J. Bonica (ed.) *Advances in Neurology* Vol. 4 (Raven Press, New York)

—— (1980) 'Introduction', *Pain* 58. 1–17

Boore, J. R. P. (1978) *Prescription for Recovery. The Effect of Preoperative Preparation of Surgical Patients on Postoperative Stress, Recovery and Infection* (Royal College of Nursing, London)

Boore, J. R. P., Champion, R. and Ferguson, M. (1987) *Nursing the Physically Ill Adult: A Textbook of Medical-Surgical Nursing* (Churchill Livingstone, Edinburgh)

Botney, M. and Fields, H. I. (1983) 'Amitriptyline potentiates morphine analgesia by a direct action on the central nervous system', *Ann. Neurol.* 13. 160–164

Bouckoms, A. J. (1994) 'Limbic surgery for pain', in P D Wall and R Melzack (eds) *Textbook of Pain* 3rd edn (Churchill Livingstone, Edinburgh)

Bourne, L. E., Dominowski, R. L. and Loftus, E. F. (1979) *Cognitive Processes* (Prentice-Hall, Englewood Cliffs NJ)

Bowers, K. (1968) 'Pain, anxiety and perceived control', *Journal of Consulting and Clinical Psychology* 32. 596–602

Braine, M. D. S., Reiser, B. J. and Rumain, B. (1984) 'Some empirical justification for a theory of natural propositional logic', in G. H. Bower (ed.) *The Psychology of Learning and Motivation* Vol. 18 (Academic Press, New York)

Breitbart, P., Passik, S. D. and Rosenfield, B. (1994) 'Psychiatric and psychosocial aspects of cancer pain', in P. D. Wall and R. Melzack (eds) *Textbook of Pain* 3rd edn (Churchill Livingstone, Edinburgh)

Brena, S. F. and Chapman, S. L. (1983) *Management of the Patient with Chronic Pain* (Medical and Scientific Books, New York)

—— (1985) 'Acute versus chronic pain states: the Learned Pain Syndrome', *Clinics in Anesthesiology* 3. 41–55

Brewster, A. B. (1982) 'Chronically ill hospitalised children's concepts of their illness', *Pediatrics* 69. 355–362

British National Formulary (1998) *BNF* 36 September (British Medical Association, London. Royal Pharmaceutical Society of Great Britain, London)

Brooking, J. (1986) 'Patient and family participation in nursing care: the development of a nursing process measuring scale' (Ph.D. Thesis, King's College, London)

Broome, M. E., Lillis, P. and Smith, M. C. (1989) 'Pain interventions with children: a meta-analysis of research', *Nursing Research* 38. 3

Brown, J. D. and Rogers, R. J. (1991) 'Self serving attributions. The role of physiological arousal', *Personality and Social Psychology Bulletin* 17. 501–506

Brown, L. (1987) 'Physiological responses to cutaneous pain in neonates', *Neonat. Network* 6. 18–22

Burns, J. W., Johnson, B. J., Mahoney, N., Devine, J. and Pawl, R. (1996) 'Anger management style, hostility and spouse responses: gender differences in predictors of adjustment among chronic pain patients', *Pain* 64. 445–453

Burton, R. (1991) 'Leisure and quality of life. Themes and issues', *Leisure Studies Association* 42

Calman, M. and Johnson, B. (1985) 'Health, health risks and inequalities', *Sociology of Health and Illness* 17

Calvillo, E. R. and Flaskerud, J. H. (1993) 'Evaluation of the pain response by Mexican American and Anglo American women and their nurses', *Journal of Advanced Nursing* 18. 451–459

Camp-Sorrell, D. and O'Sullivan, P. (1987) 'Comparison of surgical and oncology patients' descriptions of pain and nurses' documentation of pain assessment', *Journal of Advanced Nursing* 12. 593–598

—— (1991) 'Effects of continuing education: pain assessment and documentation', *Cancer Nursing* 14. 49–54

Campbell, A. (1987) *Acupuncture: The Modern Scientific Approach* (Faber and Faber, London)

Campbell, D. T. and Stanley, J. C. (1966) *Experiments and Quasi Experimental Designs for Research* (Rand McNally Co., Chicago)

Cannon, W. B. (1929) *Bodily Changes in Pain, Hunger, Fear and Rage* (Appleton, New York)

Carr, E. (1990) 'Postoperative pain patients' expectations and experiences', *Journal of Advanced Nursing* 15. 89–100

—— (1997) 'Managing postoperative pain: problems and solutions', in V. N. Thomas (ed.) *Pain: Its Nature and Management* (Baillière Tindall, London)

Carr, E. and Thomas, V. N. (1997) 'Ethical issues in pain management', in V. N. Thomas (ed.) *Pain: Its Nature and Management* (Baillière Tindall, London)

Carroll, D. (1993) 'Pain assessment', in D. Carroll and D. Bowsher (eds) *Pain: Management and Nursing Care* (Butterworth-Heinemann, Oxford)

Carroll, D. and Bowsher, D. (eds) (1993) *Pain: Management and Nursing Care* (Butterworth-Heinemann, Oxford)

Carroll, D. and Seers, K. (1998) 'Relaxation for the relief of chronic pain: a systematic review', *Journal of Advanced Nursing* 27. 476–487

Carson, M. G. and Mitchell, G. J. (1998) 'The experience of living with persistent pain', *Journal of Advanced Nursing* 28. 6. 1,242–1,248

Carter, B. (1994) *Child and Infant Pain. Principles of Nursing Care and Management* (Stanley Thornes, London)

Case, R. (1985) *Intellectual Development – Birth to Adulthood* (Academic Press, New York)

—— (1992) 'Neo-Piagetian theories of child development', in R. J. Sternberg and C. A. Berg *Intellectual Development* (Cambridge University Press, New York)

Casey, K. L. (1980) 'Reticular formation and pain: toward a unifying concept', in J. J. Bonica (ed.) *Pain* (Raven Press, New York)

Casey, K. L., Keene, J. J. and Morrow, T. (1974) 'Bulboreticular and medical thalamic unit activity in relation to aversive behaviour and pain', in J. J. Bonica (ed.) *Pain Advances in Neurology* (Raven Press, New York)

Cassel, E. J. (1991) *The Nature of Suffering and the Goals of Medicine* (Oxford University Press, Oxford)

Chadwick, R. and Tadd, W. (1992) *Ethics and Nursing Practice: A Case Study Approach* (Macmillan Education, Oxford)

Cherny, N. I. and Portenoy, R. K. (1994) 'Cancer pain: principles of assessment and syndromes', in P. D. Wall and R. Melzack (eds) *Textbook of Pain* 3rd edn (Churchill Livingstone, Edinburgh)

Ciccone, D. S. and Grzesiak, R. C. (1984) 'Cognitive dimensions of chronic pain', *Social Science and Medicine* 19. 12. 1,339–1,345

—— (1988) 'Cognitive theory: an overview of theory and practice', in N. Lynch and S. Vasudevan (eds) *Persistent Pain: Psychological Assessment and Intervention* (Kluwer Academic Publishers, Boston MA)

Clark, A. (1989) *Microcognition: Philosophy, Cognitive Science, and Parallel Distributed Processing* (MIT Press, Cambridge)

Clark, W. C. and Clark, S. B. (1980) 'Pain responses in Nepalese porters', *Science* 209. 410–412

Clifford, B. R., Bunter, B. and McAleer, J. L. (1995) *Television and Children* (Erlbaum, Hillsdale NJ)

Closs, S. (1990) 'An exploratory analysis of nurses' provision of postoperative analgesic drugs', *Journal of Advanced Nursing* 15. 42–49

—— (1996) 'Pain and elderly patients: a survey of nurses' knowledge and experiences', *Journal of Advanced Nursing* 23. 2. 237–242

Cohen, F. (1987) 'Measurement of coping', in S. V. Kaol and C. L. Cooper (eds) *Stress and Health: Issues in Health Methodology* (John Wiley and Sons, New York)

Collins, A. M. and Quillan, M. R. (1970) 'Does category size affect categorisation time?', *Journal of Verbal Learning and Verbal Behaviour* 9. 432–438

—— (1972) 'Experiments on semantic memory and language comprehension', in L. W. Gregg (ed.) *Cognition and Learning and Memory* (John Wiley, New York)

Contrada, R., Leventhal, H. and O'Leary, A. (1990) 'Personality and Health', in L Pervin (ed.) *Handbook of Personality: Theory and Research* (Guilford Press, New York)

Coopersmith, S. (1981) *Self-Esteem Inventory* (Consulting Psychologist Press, Palo Alto)

Copp, L. A. (1974) 'The spectrum of suffering', *American Journal of Nursing* 74. 3. 491–495

—— (1985) 'Pain ethics and negotiation of values', in *Perspectives on Pain: Recent Advances in Nursing* Vol. 11 (Churchill Livingstone, Edinburgh)

Corran, T. M., Gibson, S. J., Farrell, M. J. and Helme, R. D. (1994) 'Comparison of chronic pain experiences between young and elderly patients', in G. F. Gebhart, D. L. Hammond and T. S. Jensen (eds) *Progress in Pain Research and Management: Proceedings of the 7th World Congress on Pain* (IASP Press, Seattle)

Cousins, M. J. (1994) 'Acute and postoperative pain', in P. D. Wall and R. Melzack (eds) *Textbook of Pain* 3rd edn (Churchill Livingstone, Edinburgh)

Cousins, M. J. and Bridenbaugh, P. O. (1987) *Neural Blockade* (Lippincott, Philadelphia)

Craig, K. D. (1978) 'Social modelling influences on pain', in R. A. Sternbach (ed.) *The Psychology of Pain* (Raven Press, New York)

Craig, K. D., McMahon, R. J., Morison, J. D. and Zaskow, C. (1984) 'Developmental changes in infant pain expression during immunisation injections', *Social Science and Medicine* 19. 1331–1337

CSAG (1994) *Back Pain Report of a CSAG Committee on Back Pain* (Clinical Standards Advisory Group, HMSO, London)

Cummings, E. A., Reid, G. J., Finley, G. A., McGrath, P. J. and Ritchie, J. A. (1996) 'Prevalence and source of pain in pediatric inpatients', *Pain* 68. 25–31

Dahlstrom, B., Bolme, P., Feychting, H., Noack, G. and Paalzow, L. (1979) 'Morphine kinetics in children', *Clinical Pharmacology and Therapeutics* 26. 354–365

Dalton, J. A. (1989) 'Nurses' perceptions of their pain assessment skills, pain management practices and attitudes towards pain', *Oncology Nursing Forum* 16. 2. 225–231

D'Apolita, K. (1984) 'The neonate's response to pain', *Maternal Child Nursing* 9. 256–257

Darbyshire, P. (1993) 'Parents, nurses and paediatric nursing: a critical review', *Journal of Advanced Nursing* 18. 1,670–1,680

Davies, C. (1983) 'Professionals in bureaucracies: the conflict thesis revisited', in R. Dingwall and P. Lewis (eds) *The Sociology of the Professions: Lawyers, Doctors and Others* (Macmillan, London)

Davies, S. and Riches, L. (1995) 'Healing touch?', *Nursing Times* 91. 25. 42–43

Davis, B. D. (1981) 'Social skills in nursing', in M. I. Argyle (ed.) *Social Skills and Health* (Methuen, London)

—— (1984a) *Pre-operative Information Giving and Patients' Post-operative Outcomes: An Implementation Study* Report prepared for the Scottish Home and Health Department (Nursing Research Unit, University of Edinburgh, Department of Nursing Studies)

—— (1984b) *The Study of Patients' Fears and Worries* Report prepared for the Scottish Home and Health Department (Nursing Research Unit, University of Edinburgh, Department of Nursing Studies)

—— (1984c) 'What is the nurses' perception of patient?', in S. Skevington (ed.) *Understanding Nurses: The Social Psychology of Nursing* (Wiley, Chichester)

—— (1990) 'Empathy in transcultural nursing practice', in R. C. McKay, J. R. Hughes and E. J. Carver (eds) *Empathy in the Helping Relationship* (Springer Publishing Company, New York)

—— (1998) 'Cultural dimensions of pain', in B. Carter (ed.) *Perspectives on Pain* (Arnold, London)

Davis, B. D. and Dreliozi, A. (1996) 'Cognitive development and the prevention of pain in children', paper presented at the 4th European Conference on Pain Research, Amsterdam. Proceedings in *Dolor, Investigacions, Clinica and Terapeutica* 11 Supp. 1

Davis, B. D., Billings, J. R. and Ryland, R. K. (1994) 'Evaluation of nursing process documentation', *Journal of Advanced Nursing* 19. 960–968

Davis, B. D., Cowley, S. A. and Ryland, R. K. (1996) 'The effects of terminal illness on patients and their carers', *Journal of Advanced Nursing* 23. 3. 512–520

Davis, P. (1988a) 'Changing nursing practice for more effective control of postoperative pain through a staff initiated educational programme', *Nurse Education Today* 8. 325–331

——(1988b) *Aromatherapy: An A–Z* (C. W. Daniel, Saffron Walden)

Davis, P. and Seers, K. (1991) 'Teaching nurses about managing pain', *Nursing Standard* 5. 52. 30–32

Davitz, J. R. and Davitz, L. J. (1981) *Influences on Patients' Pain and Psychological Distress* (Springer-Verlag, New York)

Deci, E. L. and Ryan, R. M. (1987) 'The support of autonomy and the control of behaviour', *Journal of Personality and Social Psychology* 53. 6. 1,024–1,037

De Rond, M., de Wit, R., van Dam, F., van Campen, B., den Hartog, Y., Kleivink, R., Nieweg, R., Noort, J., Wagenaar, M. and van Campen, B. (1999) 'Daily pain assessment: value for nurses and patients', *Journal of Advanced Nursing* 29. 2. 436–444

De Veber, L. L. (1986) 'Cancer pain in children', paper presented at the 6th World Congress on the Terminally Ill, Montreal

De Wit, R., van Dam, F., Zandbelt, L., van Buuren, A., van der Heijden, K., Leenhouts, G. and Loonstra, S. (1997) 'A pain education program for chronic cancer pain patients: follow up results from a randomised control trial', *Pain* 73. 55–69

De Wit, R., van Dam, F., Hanneman, M., Zandbelt, L., van Buuren, A., van der Heijden, K., Leenhouts, G., Loonstra, S. and Abu-Saad, H. H. (1999) 'Evaluation of the use of a pain diary in chronic cancer pain patients at home', *Pain* 79. 89–99

Diamond, A. W. and Coniam, S. W. (1991) *The Management of Chronic Pain* (Oxford University Press, Oxford)

Doan, B. D. and Wadden, N. P. (1989) 'Relationships between depressive symptoms and descriptions of chronic pain', *Pain* 36. 1. 75–84

Doehring, K. M. (1989) 'Relieving pain through touch', *Advancing Clinical Care* Sept., 32–33

Dollard, J. and Miller, N. (1950) *Personality and Psychotherapy: An Analysis in Terms of Learning, Thinking and Culture* (McGraw-Hill, New York)

Donaldson, M. (1978) *Children's Minds* (Fontana Collins, London)

Donovan, M., Dillon, P. and McGuire, L. (1987) 'Incidence and characteristics of pain in a sample of medical-surgical inpatients', *Pain* 30. 69–78

Doody, S. B., Smith, C. and Webb, J. (1991) 'Nonpharmacologic interventions for pain management', *Critical Care Nursing Clinics of North America* 3. 1. 69–75

Doyle, D. (1986) 'Domiciliary care – a doctor's view', in *International Symposium on Pain Control* (Royal Society of Medicine)

Duff, R. S. and Hollingshead, A. B. (1968) *Sickness and Society* (Harper and Row, New York)

Edgar, L. (1993) 'The psychological aspects of pain', in D. Carroll and D. Bowsher (eds) *Pain: Management and Nursing Care* (Butterworth-Heinemann, Oxford)

Ekman, P. (1992) 'Facial expressions of emotion: new findings, new questions', *Psychological Science* 3. 34–38

Ekman, P. and Friesen, W. V. (1969) 'The repertoire of nonverbal behaviour: categories, origins, usage and coding', *Semiotica* 1. 49–98

Ekman, P., Levenson, R. W. and Friesen, W. V. (1983) 'Autonomic nervous system activity distinguishes among emotions', *Science* 221. 1,208–1,210

Eland, J. M. (1974) 'Children's communication of pain' (Master's Thesis, University of Iowa IA)

—— (1981) 'Minimising pain associated with prekindergarten intramuscular injections', *Issues in Comprehensive Paediatric Nursing* 5. 361–372

—— (1985) 'The child who is hurting', *Seminars in Oncology Nursing* 1. 116–122

—— (1988) 'Persistence of pain research: one nurse researcher's efforts', *Recent Advances in Nursing* 21. 43–62

—— (1993) 'The use of TENS with children', in N. L. Schechter, C. B. Berde and M. Yaster (eds) *Pain in Infants, Children and Adolescents* (Williams and Watkins, Baltimore)

Eland, J. M. and Anderson, J. E. (1977) 'The experience of pain in children', in A. K. Jacox (ed.) *Pain: A Sourcebook for Nurses and Other Health Professionals* (Little, Brown, Boston)

Elton, D., Stuart, G. V. and Burrows, G. D. (1978) 'Self-esteem and chronic pain', *Journal of Psychosomatic Research* 22. 25–30

Engel, G. (1959) 'Psychogenic pain and the pain prone disorder', *American Journal of Psychiatry* 26. 899–918

Epstein, A. (1982) 'Instinct and motivation as explanations for complex behaviour', in D. W. Pfaff (ed.) *The Physiological Mechanisms of Motivation* (Springer, New York)

Epstein, N. and Bishop, D. (1981) 'Problem-centred systems therapy for the family', in A. Gurman and D. Kniskern (eds) *Handbook of Family Therapy* (Brunner/Mazel, New York)

Eriksson, M. B. E., Sjolund, B. H. and Nielzen, S. (1979) 'Long term results of peripheral conditioning stimulation as an analgesia measure in chronic pain', *Pain* 6. 335–347

Ernst, E. and Fialka, V. (1994) 'Ice freezes pain? A review of the clinical effectiveness of analgesic cold therapy', *Journal of Pain and Symptom Management* 9. 1. 56–59

Escobar, P. L. (1985) 'Management of chronic pain', *Nurse Practitioner* 10. 1. 24–25

Evans, J. (1992) 'The nursing management of postoperative pain: policies, politics and strategies', *Journal of Clinical Nursing* 1. 226

Evers, H. K. (1981) 'Tender loving care? Patients and nurses in geriatric wards', in L. A. Copp (ed.) *Care of the Ageing* (Churchill Livingstone, Edinburgh)

Fabrega, H. and Tyma, S. (1976) 'Culture, language and the shaping of illness: an illustration based on pain', *Journal of Psychosomatic Research* 20. 323–337

Fagerhaugh, S. (1974) 'Pain expression on a burn care unit', *Nursing Outlook* 22. 645–650

Fagerhaugh, S. and Strauss, A. (1977) *Politics of Pain Management: Staff–Patient Interaction* (Addison-Wesley, California)

Faymonville, M. E., Mambourg, P. H., Joris, J., Vrijens, B., Fissette, J., Albert, A. and Lamy, M. (1997) 'Psychological approaches during conscious sedation. Hypnosis versus stress reducing strategies: a prospective randomised study', *Pain* 73. 361–367

Fellner, C. H. (1971) 'Alterations in pain perceptions of multiple sensory modality stimulation', *Psychosomatics* 12. 313–315

Ferrell, B. R., Eberts, M. T., McCaffery, M. and Grant, M. (1991) 'Clinical decision making and pain', *Cancer Nursing* 14. 6. 289–297

Ferrel-Torry, A. and Glick, O. (1993) 'The use of therapeutic massage as a nursing intervention to modify anxiety and the perception of cancer pain', *Cancer Nursing* 16. 2. 93–101

Festinger, L. (1954) 'A theory of social comparison processes', *Human Relations* 7. 117–140

Fields, H. (ed.) (1995) *Core Curriculum for Professional Education in Pain* (IASP, Seattle)

Fields, H. L. and Basbaum, A. I. (1994) 'Central nervous system mechanisms of pain modulation', in P. D. Wall and R. Melzack (eds) *Textbook of Pain* 3rd edn (Churchill Livingstone, Edinburgh)

Findlay, J. W. A., Jones, E. C., Butz, R. F. and Welch, R. M. (1978) 'Plasma codeine and morphine concentrations after therapeutic doses of codeine containing analgesics', *Clinical Pharmacology and Therapeutics* 24. 60–68

Fischer, K. W., Shaver, P. R. and Carnochan, P. (1990) 'How emotions develop and how they organise development', *Cognition and Emotion* 4. 81–127

Fisher, R. A. (1991) 'Introduction: palliative care – a rediscovery', in J. Penson and R. Fisher (eds) *Palliative Care for People with Cancer: A Guide for Nurses* (Edward Arnold, London)

Fishman, B. and Loscalzo, M. (1987) 'Cognitive behavioural interventions in management of cancer pain: principles and applications', *Medical Clinics of North America* 71. 2. 271–287

Fitton, F. and Ascherson, H. W. K. (1979) *The Doctor–Patient Relationship in General Practice* (HMSO, London)

Flor, H., Turk, D. and Scholtz, O. (1987) 'Impact of chronic pain on the spouse: marital, emotional and physical consequences', *Journal Psychosomatic Research* 31. 63–72

Follick, M. J., Ahern, D. K. and Laser-Wolston, N. (1984) 'Evaluation of a daily activity diary for chronic pain patients', *Pain* 19. 373–382

Fordham, M. and Dunn, V. (1994) *Alongside the Person in Pain* (Baillière Tindall, London)

Fordyce, W. E. (1976) *Behavioural Methods for Chronic Pain and Illness* (C. V. Mosby, St Louis)

—— (1984) 'Behavioural science and chronic pain', *Postgraduate Medical Journal* 60. 865–868

Fosburg, M. T. and Crone, R. K. (1983) 'Nitrous oxide analgesia for refractory pain in the terminally ill', *Journal of the American Medical Association* 250. 511–513

Fothergill-Bourbonnais, F. and Wilson-Barnett, J. (1992) 'A comparative study of intensive therapy unit hospice nurses' knowledge on pain management', *Journal of Advanced Nursing* 17. 362–372

Fowler-Kerry, S. and Lander, J. R. (1987) 'Management of injection pain in children', *Pain* 30. 169–175

Franck, L. S. (1986) 'A new method to quantitatively describe pain behaviour in infants', *Nursing Research* 35. 28–31

Franke, A. L., Garssen, B. and Abu-Saad, H. H. (1996) 'Continuing pain education in nursing: a literature review', *International Journal of Nursing Studies* 33. 5. 567–578

Fransella, F. (1995) *George Kelly* (Sage, London)

Frazier, P. A. (1990) 'Victim attributions and post-rape trauma', *Journal of Personality and Social Psychology* 59. 293–311

French, J. R. P. and Raven, B. (1959) 'The bases of social power', in D Cartwright (ed.) *Studies in Social Power* (University of Michigan Press, Ann Arbor)

—— (1968) 'The bases of social power', in D. Cartwright and A. Zander (eds) *Group Dynamics: Research and Theory* (Harper and Row, New York)

Frost, F. A., Jessen, B. and Siggaard Andersen, J. (1980) 'A control double blind comparison of mepivacaine injection versus saline injection for myofascial pain', *Lancet* 8. 499–501

Fuller, B. F., Yoshiyuki, H. and Conner, D. (1994) 'Vocal measures in infant pain', in S. G. Funk, E. M. Tornquist, M. T. Champagne, L. A. Copp and R. A. Weise (eds) *Management of Pain, Fatigue and Nausea* (Macmillan Press, Basingstoke)

Gadish, H. S., Gonzalez, J. L. and Hayes, J. S. (1988) 'Factors affecting nurses' decisions to administer pediatric medication postoperatively', *Pediatric Nursing* 3. 6. 383–389

Gaffney, A. (1988) 'How children describe pain: a study of words and analogies used by 5–14-year-olds', in R Dubner, G. F. Gebhart and M. Bond (eds) *The 5th World Congress of Pain* (Elsevier, Amsterdam)

Gaffney, A. and Dunne, E. A. (1986) 'Developmental aspects of children's definition of pain', *Pain* 26. 105–117

—— (1987) 'Children's understanding of the causality of pain', *Pain* 29. 91–104

Gagliese, L. and Melzack, R. (1997) 'Chronic pain in elderly people', *Pain* 70. 3–14

Gale, A. (ed.) (1986) *Physiological Correlates of Human Behaviour* (Academic Press, New York)

Gallagher, R., Rauh, V., Haugh, L. and Mithons, P. (1989) 'Determinants of return to work among low back pain patients', *Pain* 39. 55–68

Gattuso, S. M., Litt, M. D. and Fitzgerald, T. E. (1992) 'Coping with gastro-intestinal endoscopy, self-efficacy enhancement and coping style', *Journal of Consulting and Clinical Psychology* 60. 133–139

Gauld, A. (1986) 'Reflections on mesmeric analgesia', *British Journal of Experimental and Clinical Hypnosis* 5. 17–24

Gautrey, J. P., Jolivet, A., Veilh, J. P. and Guillemin, R. (1977) 'Presence of immunoassayable beta endorphins in human amniotic fluid: elevation in cases of foetal distress', *Am. Journal of Obstetrics and Gynaecology* 121. 211–212

Gazda, G. M., Childers, W. C. and Brooks, D. K., Jr (1987) *Foundations of Counselling and Human Services* (McGraw-Hill, New York)

Geisser, M. E., Robinson, M. E., Keefe, F. J. and Weiner, M. L. (1994) 'Catastrophising, depression and the sensory, affective and evaluative aspects of chronic pain', *Pain* 59. 79–83

Gilbert, G. N. and Mulkay, M. (1984) *Opening Pandora's Box: A Sociological Analysis of Scientists' Discourse* (Cambridge University Press, Cambridge)

Gill, L. J., Shand, P. A. X., Fuggle, P., Dugan, B. and Davies, S. C. (1997) 'Pain assessment for children with sickle cell disease: improved validity of diary keeping versus interview ratings', *British Journal of Health Psychology* 2. 131–140

Gloor, P. (1978) 'Inputs and outputs of the amygdala: what the amygdala is trying to tell the rest of the brain', in K. E. Livingstone and D. Hornykiewicz (eds) *Limbic Mechanisms* (Plenum Press, New York)

Goffman, E. (1974) *Frame Analysis: An Essay on the Organisation of Experience* (Penguin, Harmondsworth)

Goldberg, R. T., Pachas, W. N. and Keith, D. (1999) 'Relationship between traumatic events in childhood and chronic pain', *Disability and Rehabilitation* 21. 1. 23–30

Goldman, A. and Lloyd-Thomas, A. R. (1991) 'Pain management in children', *British Medical Bulletin* 47. 676–689

Goldschneider, K. R. (1998) 'Long-term consequences of pain in infancy', *IASP Newsletter* July/August

Goldsheider, A. (1894) *Über den Schmerz in physiologischer und klinischer Hinsicht* (Hirschwald, Berlin)

Gonzalez, J. C., Routh, D. K. and Armstrong, F. D. (1993) 'Differential medication of child versus adult postoperative patients: the effects of nurses' assumptions', *Children's Health Care* 22. 47–59

Gray, J. A. (1990) 'Brain systems that medicate both emotion and cognition', *Cognition and Emotion* 4. 269–288

Green, S. (1987) *Physiological Psychology: An Introduction* (Routledge and Kegan Paul, London)

Griepp, M. E. (1992) 'Griepp's model of ethical decision making', *Journal of Advanced Nursing* 17. 734–738

Grunau, R. V. E. and Craig, K. D. (1987) 'Pain expression in neonates: facial action and crying', *Pain* 28. 395–410

—— (1990) 'Facial activity as a measure of neonatal pain expression', in D. C. Tyler and E. J. Krane (eds) *Advances in Pain Research and Therapy*, Vol. 15 *Pediatric Pain* (Raven Press, New York)

Grunau, R. E., Oberlander, T., Holstii, L. and Whitfield, M. F. (1998) 'Bedside application of the Neonatal Facial Coding System in pain assessment of premature neonates', *Pain* 76. 277–286

Grunau, R. E., Whitfield, M. F. and Petrie, J. H. (1994) 'Pain sensitivity and temperament in extremely low birth-weight premature toddlers and preterm and full term controls', *Pain* 58. 341–346

Hadjistavropoulos, H. D., Craig, K. D., Grunau, R. E. and Whitfield, M. F. (1997) 'Judging pain in infants: behavioural, contextual and developmental determinants', *Pain* 73. 319–324

Haldeman, S. (1994) 'Manipulation and massage for the relief of back pain', in P. D. Wall and R. Melzack (eds) *Textbook of Pain* 3rd edn (Churchill Livingstone, Edinburgh)

Haley, W. E., Turner, J. A. and Romano, J. M. (1985) 'Depression in chronic pain patients: relation to pain activity and sex differences', *Pain* 23. 337–343

Hall, K. R. L. and Stride, E. (1954) 'The varying response to pain in psychiatric disorders: a study in abnormal psychology', *British Journal of Medical Psychology* 27. 48–60

Halperin, D. L., Koren, G. and Attias, D. (1989) 'Topical skin anesthesia for venous subcutaneous drug reservoir and lumbar punctures in children', *Pediatrics* 84. 281–284

Hamers, J. P. H., Abu Saad, H. H., Halfens, R. J. G. and Schumacher, J. N. M. (1994) 'Factors influencing nurses' pain assessment and interventions in children', *Journal of Advanced Nursing* 20. 853–860

Hamers, J. P. H., Abu Saad, H. H., van der Hout, M. A. and Halfens, R. J. G. (1998) 'Are children given insufficient pain relieving medication postoperatively?', *Journal of Advanced Nursing* 27. 37–44

Hanks, G. W., de Conno, F., Hanna, M., McQuay, H. J., Mercadante, S., Meynadier, J., Poulain, P. and Roca, I. Casas (1996) 'Morphine in cancer pain: modes of administration. Expert working group of the European Association for Palliative Care', *British Medical Journal* 312. 823–826

Hanks, G. W., Hoskin, P. J. and Aherne, G. W. (1987) 'Explanation for potency of repeated oral doses of morphine?', *Lancet* 2. 723–725

Hardy, J. D., Wolff, H. G. and Goodell, H. (1952) *Pain Sensations and Reactions* (Williams and Wilkins, Baltimore)

Hardy, L. (1988) 'The inverted U hypothesis: a catastrophe for sport psychology', paper presented at the British Psychological Society Annual Conference, Leeds

Harre, R. (1979) *Social Being* (Basil Blackwell, Oxford)

Hawthorn, J. and Redmond, K. (1998) *Pain: Causes and Management* (Blackwell, Oxford)

Hayes, N. (1994) *Foundations of Psychology: An Introductory Text* (Routledge, London)

Haythornthwaite, J. A., Menefee, L., Heinberg, L. J. and Clark, M. R. (1998) 'Pain coping strategies predict perceived control over pain', *Pain* 77. 33–39

Hayward, J. (1975) *Information. A Prescription Against Pain* (Royal College of Nursing, London)

Hayward, S. (1996) *Biopsychology. Physiological Psychology. Introductory Psychology* (Macmillan, London)

Hazinski, M. (1984) 'Children are different', in M Hazinski (ed.) *Nursing Care of the Critically Ill Child* (Mosby, St Louis)

Heath, M. L. (1993) 'The use of pharmacology in pain management', in V. N. Thomas (ed.) *Pain: Its Nature and Management* (Baillière Tindall, London)

Heaven, C. M. and Maguire, P. (1996) 'Training hospice nurses to elicit patient concerns', *Journal of Advanced Nursing* 23. 280–286

Hebb, D. O. (1955) 'Drives and the conceptual nervous system', *Psychological Review* 62. 243–254

Heider, F. (1958) *The Psychology of Interpersonal Relations* (John Wiley, New York)

Helman, C. G. (1994) *Culture, Health and Illness* 3rd edn (Butterworth-Heinemann, Oxford)

Herbert, C. (1998) 'Nursing considerations: the role of non-pharmacological interventions for acute traumatic pain in the accident and emergency department', BN dissertation School of Nursing, University of Wales College of Medicine, Cardiff

Hermann, C., Kim, M. and Blanchard, E. B. (1995) 'Behavioural and prophylactic pharmacological intervention studies of pediatric migraine: an exploratory meta-analysis', *Pain* 60. 239–256

Hester, N. K. (1979) 'The pre-operation child's reaction to immunisation', *Nursing Research* 28. 250–255

Hester, N. K., Foster, R. and Kristiensen, K. (1990) 'Measurement of pain in children: generalisability and validity of the pain ladder and the poker chip tool', in D. C. Tyler and E. J. Krane (eds) *Advances in Pain Research and Therapy: Pediatric Pain* (Raven Press, New York)

Hilgard, E. R. and Hilgard, J. R. (1983) *Hypnosis in the Relief of Pain* (William Kaufman, Los Altos CA)

Hilgard, J. R. and LeBaron, S. (1984) *Hypnotherapy of Pain in Children with Cancer* (William Kaufman, Los Altos CA)

Hill, H. E., Kornetsky, C. H., Flanary, H. G. and Wikler, A. (1952) 'Effects of anxiety and morphine on discrimination of intensities of painful stimuli', *Journal of Clinical Investigation* 31. 473–480

Hollingworth, H. (1995) 'Nurses' assessment and management of pain at wound dressing changes', *Journal of Wound Care* 4. 2. 77–83

Horn, S. and Munafo, M. (1997) *Pain: Theory, Research and Intervention* (Open University Press, Buckingham)

Horrigan, C. (1993) 'Alternative nursing interventions', in D. Carroll and D. Bowsher (1993) *Pain: Management and Nursing Care* (Butterworth-Heinemann, Oxford)

Hudgens, A. (1979) 'Family oriented treatment of chronic pain', *Journal of Marital and Family Therapy* 5. 67–76

Hughes, J., Smith, T. W., Kosterlitz, H. W., Fothergill, L. A., Morgan, B. A. and Morris, H. R. (1975) 'Identification of two related pentapeptides from the brain with potent opiate agonist activity', *Nature* 58. 577–579

Hull, C. (1952) *A Behaviour System* (Yale University Press, New Haven)

Hunt, J. M. and Marks-Maran, D. J. (1986) *Nursing Care Plans: The Nursing Process at Work* (H. M. & M. Publishers Ltd, London)

Hunt, S. and McKenna, S. (1992) 'Do we need measure other than QALY's?', in A. H. Hopkins (ed.) *Measures of the Quality of Life and the Uses to Which Such Measures May Be Put* (Royal College of Physicians, London)

Hunter, D. (1993) 'Acute pain', in D. Carroll and D. Bowsher (eds) *Pain: Management and Nursing Care* (Butterworth-Heinemann, Oxford)

IASP Sub-committee on Taxonomy (1979) 'Pain terms: a list with definitions and notes on usage', *Pain* 6. 249–252

IASP (1992) 'Management of acute pain: a practical guide', in L. B. Ready (ed.) *Task Force on Acute Pain* (IASP Press, Seattle)

—— (1995) 'Core curriculum for professional education in pain', in H. L. Fields (ed.) *A Report of the Task Force on Professional Education of the International Association for the Study of Pain* (IASP Press, Seattle)

Illich, I. (1976) *Limits to Medicine* (Marion Boyars, London)

Inturrisi, C. E. and Hanks, G. (1993) 'Opioid analgesic therapy', in D. Doyle, G. W. C. Hanks and N. MacDonald (eds) *Oxford Textbook of Palliative Medicine* (Oxford Medical Publications, Oxford)

Ischia, S., Ischia, S., Luzzani, A., Toscano, D. and Steele, A. (1985) 'Results up to death in the treatment of persistent cervico-thoracic (Pancoast) and thoracic malignant pain by unilateral percutaneous cervical cordotomy', *Pain* 21. 339–355

Jadad, A. R., Moore, R. A. and Carroll, D. (1996) 'Assessing the quality of reports of randomised controlled clinical trials: is blinding necessary?', *Controlled Clinical Trials* 17. 1–12

Jaffe, J. H. (1975) 'Drug addiction and drug abuse', in L. S. Goodman and M. Gilman (eds) *The Pharmacological Basis of Therapeutics* 5th edn (Macmillan, Basingstoke)

Jeffrey, R. (1979) 'Normal rubbish: deviant patients in casualty departments', *Sociology of Health and Illness* 1. 90–107

Jensen, I. B. and Bodin, L. (1998) 'Multimodal cognitive-behavioural treatment for workers with chronic spinal pain: a matched cohort study with an 18-month follow-up', *Pain* 76. 35–44

Jensen, T. S., Krebs, B., Nielson, J. and Rasmussen, P. (1985) 'Immediate and long-term phantom limb pain in amputees: incidence, clinical characteristics and relationship to pre-amputation limb pain', *Pain* 21. 267–278

Jensen, T., Turner, J. A., Hallin, Z. W. (eds) (1997) 'Preface', *Proceedings of the 8th World Congress on Pain* (IASP Press, Seattle)

Jessup, B. A. and Gallegos, X. (1994) 'Relaxation and biofeedback', in P. D. Wall and R. Melzack (eds) *Textbook of Pain* 3rd edn (Churchill Livingstone, Edinburgh)

Johnson, J. and Vogele, C. (1993) 'Benefits of psychological preparations for surgery: an analysis', *Annals of Behavioural Medicine* 15 September

Johnson, J. E., Rice, V. H., Fuller, S. S. and Endress, M. P. (1978) 'Sensory information, instruction in a coping strategy and recovery from surgery', *Research in Nursing and Health* 1. 1. 4–17

Johnson, M. H., Breakwell, G., Douglas, W. and Humphries, S. (1998) 'The effects of imagery and sensory detection distractors on different measures of pain: how does distraction work?', *British Journal of Clinical Psychology* 37. 141–154

Johnson, M. I., Ashton, C. H. and Thompson, J. W. (1991) 'An in-depth study of long-term users of transcutaneous electrical nerve stimulation (TENS). Implications for clinical use of TENS', *Pain* 44. 221–229

Johnson-Laird, P. N. (1983) 'Ninth Bartlett memorial lecture: thinking as a skill', *Quarterly Journal of Experimental Psychology* 34. 1–29

Johnston, C. C. and Strada, M. E. (1986) 'Acute pain response in infants: a multidimensional description', *Pain* 24. 373–382

Johnston, M. (1980) 'Anxiety in surgical patients', *Psychological Medicine* 10. 145–152

Jones, A. K. P. (1997) 'Pain, its perception and pain imaging', *IASP Newsletter* May/June

Jones, E. E. and Davis, K. E. (1965) 'From acts to dispositions: the attribution process in person perception', in L. Berkowitz (ed.) *Advances in Experimental Social Psychology* Vol. 2 (Academic Press, New York)

Justins, D. (1998) 'Research and development priorities in pain management', in C. Stannard (ed.) *The Pain Society Newsletter* 1. 5. Winter (The Pain Society, London)

Kahn, W. A. (1989) 'Towards a sense of organisational humor: implications for organisational diagnosis and change', *Journal of Applied Behavioural Science* 25. 45–63

Kaiko, R. F. (1980) 'Age and morphine analgesia in cancer patients with postoperative pain', *Clinical Pharmacology and Therapeutics* 28. 823–826

Kail, R. and Bisanz, J. (1982) 'Information processing and cognitive development', in *Advances in Child Development and Behaviour* (Academic Press, New York)

Kanfer, F. H. and Seidner, M. L. (1973) 'Self-control – factors enhancing tolerance of noxious stimulation', *Journal of Personality and Social Psychology* 25. 3. 381–389

Karoly, P. and Jensen, M. P. (1987) *Multimethod Assessment of Chronic Pain* (Pergamon Press, New York)

Katz, E. R., Kelerman, J. and Ellenberg, L. (1987) 'Hypnosis in the reduction of acute pain and distress in children with cancer', *Journal of Pediatric Psychology* 12. 379–394

Katz, J. and Melzack, R. (1990) 'Pain "memories" in phantom limbs: review and clinical observations', *Pain* 43. 319–336

Keefe, F. J. (1982) 'Behavioural assessment and treatment of chronic pain: current status and future trends', *Journal of Consulting and Clinical Psychology* 50. 896–911

Keefe, F. J., Brown, G. K., Wallston, K. A. and Caldwell, D. S. (1989) 'Coping with rheumatoid arthritis pain: catastrophising as a maladaptive strategy', *Pain* 37. 51–56

Keefe, F. J., Kashikar-Zuck, S., Robinson, E., Salley, A., Beaupre, P., Caldwell, D., Baucom, D. and Haythornwaite, J. (1998) 'Pain coping strategies that predict patients' and spouses' ratings of patients' self efficacy', *Pain* 73. 191–199

Keesing, R. M. (1981) *Cultural Anthropology: A Contemporary Perspective* (Holt, Rinehart and Winston, New York)

Kelley, H. H. (1967) 'Attribution theory in social psychology', in D. L. Vine (ed.) *Nebraska Symposium on Motivation* (University of Nebraska Press, Lincoln NE)

—— (1973) 'The process of causal attribution', *American Psychologist* 28. 107–128

Kelly, G. A. (1955) *The Psychology of Personal Constructs* (Norton, New York)

—— (1991) *The Psychology of Personal Constructs* (Routledge, London)

Kelly, M. P. and May, D. (1982) 'Good and bad patients: a review of the literature and a theoretical critique', *Journal of Advanced Nursing* 7. 147–156

Kennedy, I. (1981) *The Unmasking of Medicine* (Allen and Unwin, London)

Kenner, D. J. (1994) 'A total approach to pain management', *Australian Family Physician* 23. 1,267–1,283

Kerr, F. W., Wilson, P. R. and Nijensohn, D. E. (1960) 'Acupuncture reduces the trigeminal evoked response in decerebrate cats', *Experimental Neurology* 61. 84–95

Kim, H. S., Schwartz-Barcott, D., Holter, I. M. and Lorensen, M. (1995) 'Developing a translation of the McGill Pain Questionnaire for cross-cultural comparison: an example from Norway', *Journal of Advanced Nursing* 21. 421–426

King, I. (1981) *A Theory of Nursing: Systems, Concepts, Process* (John Wiley, New York)

King, L. (1997) 'The influence of nursing expertise on the assessment of pain: a qualitative study', in V. N. Thomas (ed.) *Pain: Its Nature and Management* (Baillière Tindall, London)

Kleinman, A. (1988) *The Illness Narratives: Suffering, Healing and the Human Condition* (Basic Books, New York)

Kleinman, A., Eisenberg, L. and Good, B. (1978) 'Culture, illness and care: clinical lessons from anthropologic and cross-cultural research', *Annals of International Medicine* 88. 251–258

Knardahl, S., Elam, M., Olausson, B. and Wallin, B. G. (1998) 'Sympathetic nerve activity after acupuncture in humans', *Pain* 75. 19–25

Kohler, W. (1925) *The Mentality of Apes* (Harcourt Brace, New York)

Kosko, D. A. and Flaskerud, J. H. (1987) 'Mexican American, nurse practitioner, and lay control beliefs about cause and treatment of chest pain', *Nursing Research* 36. 4. 226–230

Koutantji, M., Pearce, S. A. and Oakley, D. (1998) 'The relationship between gender and family history of pain with current pain experience and awareness of pain in others', *Pain* 77. 25–31

Krech, D., Crutchfield, R. S. and Ballachey, E. L. (1971) *Individual in Society: A Textbook of Social Psychology* (McGraw-Hill, London)

Kruglanski, A. W., Baldwin, M. W. and Towson, M. J. (1983) 'The lay epistemic process in attribution making', in M. Hewstone (ed.) *Attribution Theory: Social and Functional Extensions* (Basil Blackwell, Oxford)

Labbe, E. L. and Williamson, D. A. (1984) 'Treatment of childhood migraine using autogenic feedback training', *Journal of Consulting and Clinical Psychology* 52. 968–976

Lalljee, M. (1981) 'Attribution theory and the analysis of explanations', in C. Antaki (ed.) *The Psychology of Ordinary Explanations of Social Behaviour* (Academic Press, London)

Lambert, W. E., Libman, E. and Poser. E. G. (1960) 'Effect of increased salience of membership group on pain tolerance', *Journal of Personality* 28. 350–357

Large, R. and Strong, J. (1997) 'The personal constructs of coping with chronic low back pain: is coping a necessary evil?', *Pain* 73. 245–252

Larsen, R. J. and Diener, E. (1987) 'Affect intensity as an individual differences characteristic: a review', *Journal of Research in Personality* 21. 1–39

Larson-Beck, S. (1991) 'The therapeutic use of music for cancer related pain', *Oncology Nursing Forum* 18. 8. 1,327–1,337

Latham, J. and Davis, B. D. (1994) 'The socio-economic impact of chronic pain', *Disability and Rehabilitation* 16

Lawrence, J., Alcock, D., McGrath, P., Kay, J., MacMurray, S. B. and Dulberg, C. (1993) 'The development of a tool to assess neonatal pain', *Neonatal Network* 12. 6. 59–66

Lazarus, R. (1980) 'Thoughts on the relations between cognition and emotion', *American Psychologist* 37. 1,019–1,024

—— (1991) 'Cognition and motivation in emotion', *American Psychologist* 46. 352–367

Lazarus, R. and Folkman, S. (1984) *Stress, Appraisal and Coping* (Springer Publications, New York)

Leavitt, F. (1985) 'Pain and deception: use of verbal pain measurement as a diagnostic aid in differentiating between clinical and simulated low back pain', *Journal of Psychosomatic Research* 29. 5. 495–505

Leavitt, F. and Sweet, B. (1986) 'Characteristics and frequency of malingering among patients with low back pain', *Pain* 25. 357–364

Le Bars, D., Dickenson, A. H. and Besson, J. M. (1983) 'Opiate analgesia and descending control systems', in J. J. Bonica *et al.* (eds) *Advances in Pain Research and Therapy* (Raven Press, New York)

Le Doux, J. E. (1986) 'The neurobiology of emotion', in J. E. Le Doux and W. Hirst (eds) *Mind and Brain: Dialogues in Cognitive Neuropsychology* (Cambridge University Press, New York)

—— (1989) 'Cognitive emotional interactions in the brain', *Cognition and Emotion* 3. 267–289

—— (1992) 'Emotional memory systems in the brain', *Behavioural Brain Research* 58. 69–79

Lefebvre, M. F. (1981) 'Cognitive distortion and cognitive errors in depressed psychiatric and low back pain patients', *Journal of Consulting and Clinical Psychology* 49. 4. 517–525

LeFort, S. M., Gray-Donald, K., Rowat, K. M. and Jeans, M. E. (1998) 'Randomised controlled trial of a community-based psychoeducation program for the self management of chronic pain', *Pain* 74. 297–306

Leininger, M. M. (ed.) (1991) *Culture Care. Diversity and Universality: A Theory of Nursing* (National League for Nursing Press, New York)

Levenson, R. W. (1992) 'Autonomic nervous system differences among emotions', *Psychological Science* 3. 23–27

Leventhal, H. (1982) 'The integration of emotion and cognition: a view from the perceptual motor theory of emotion', in M. Clarke and S. Fiske (eds) *The Seventeenth Annual Carnegie Symposium on Cognition* (Lawrence Erlbaum Associates, Hillsdale NJ)

Leventhal, H. and Mosbach, P. A. (1983) 'The perceptual-motor theory of emotion', in J. T. Cacioppo and R. E. Petty (eds) *Social Psychophysiology – A Sourcebook* (Guilford Press, New York)

Leventhal, H., Meyer, D. and Nerenz, D. (1980) 'The commonsense representation of illness danger', in S. Rachman (ed.) *Medical Psychology* Vol. 2 (Pergamon, New York)

Leventhal, H., Nerenz, D. R. and Steele, D. J. (1984) 'Illness representations and coping with health threats', in A. B. Shelley, E. Taylor and J. E. Singer (eds) *Handbook of Psychology and Health* (Lawrence Erlbaum Associates, Hillsdale NJ)

Leventhal, H., Leventhal, E. A. and Schaefer, P. (1988) 'Vigilant coping and health behaviour: a lifespan problem', unpublished manuscript

Levin, D. N., Cleeland, C. S. and Dar, R. (1985) 'Public attitudes towards cancer pain', *Cancer* 56. 2,337–2,339

Levin, D. N., Malloy, G. B. and Hyman, R. B. (1987) 'Nursing management of post-operative pain: use of relaxation techniques with female cholecystectomy patients', *Journal of Advanced Nursing* 12. 463–472

Levine, J. D. and Gordon, N. C. (1982) 'Pain in pre-lingual children and its evaluation by pain induced vocalisation', *Pain* 14. 85–93

Levine, R. M. (1999) 'Identity and illness: the effects of identity salience and frame of reference on evaluation of illness and injury', *British Journal of Health Psychology* 4. 63–80

Levy, D. (1960) 'The infant's early memory of inoculation', *Journal of Genetic Psychology* 96. 3. 46

Lewit, K. (1979) 'The needle effect in the relief of myofascial pain', *Pain* 6. 83–90

Lewith, G. and Aldridge, D. (eds) (1993) *Clinical Research Methodology for Complementary Therapies* (Hodder and Stoughton, London)

Lewith, G., Kenyon, J. and Lewis, P. (1996) *Complementary Medicine: An Integrated Approach* (Oxford University Press, Oxford)

Linton, S. (1982) 'A critical review of behavioural treatments for chronic benign pain other than headache', *British Journal of Clinical Psychology* 21. 321–327

—— (1986) 'Behavioural remediation of chronic pain: a status report', *Pain* 24. 125–141

—— (1997) 'A population-based study of the relationship between sexual abuse and back pain: establishing a link', *Pain* 73. 47–53

—— (1998) 'The socioeconomic impact of chronic back pain: is anyone benefiting?', *Pain* 75. 163–168

Linton, S. J., Larden, M. and Gillow, A. M. (1996) 'Sexual abuse and chronic musculoskeletal pain: prevalence and psychological factors', *Clinical Journal of Pain* 12. 215–221

Llewellyn, N. (1997) 'The management of children's pain', in V. N. Thomas (ed.) *Pain: Its Nature and Management* (Baillière Tindall, London)

Lorig, K., Chastain, R. L., Ung, E., Shoor, S. and Holman, H. R. (1989) 'Development and evaluation of a scale to measure perceived self-efficacy in people with arthritis', *Arthritis and Rheumatism* 32. 1. 37–44

Lundeberg, T. (1984) 'Long term results of vibratory stimulation as a pain relieving measure for chronic pain', *Pain* 20. 13–23

Lynn, A. M. and Slattery, J. T. (1987) 'Morphine pharmacokinetics in early infancy', *Anesthesiology* 66. 136–139

Lynn, B. (1977) 'Cutaneous hyperalgesia', *British Medical Bulletin* 33. 103–108

MacIntyre, D. I. and Cantrell, P. J. (1995) 'Punishment history and adult attitudes towards violence and aggression in men and women', *Social Behaviour and Personality* 23. 23–28

Mackintosh, C. and Bowles, S. (1997) 'Evaluation of a nurse-led acute pain service. Can clinical nurse specialists make a difference?', *Journal of Advanced Nursing* 25. 30–37

Manchini, V. S., Peterson, R. A. and Maruta, T. (1988) 'Changes in perception of illness and psychosocial adjustment-findings of a pain management program', *Clinical Journal of Pain* 4. 249–256

Marks, R. M. and Sachar, E. J. (1973) 'Undertreatment of medical inpatients with narcotic analgesia', *Annals of Internal Medicine* 78. 173–181

Maruta, T. and Osborne, D. (1978) 'Sexual activity in chronic pain patients', *Psychosomatics* 20. 241–248

Maruta, T., Malinchoc, M., Offord, K. and Colligan, R. C. (1998) 'Status of patients with chronic pain 13 years after treatment in a pain management center', *Pain* 74. 199–204

Maslow, A. H. (1954) *Motivation and Personality* 2nd edn 1970 (Harper and Row, New York)

Mather, L. and Mackie, J. (1983) 'The incidence of postoperative pain in children', *Pain* 5. 271–282

Mayer, D. J., Price, D. D. and Raffii, A. (1976) 'Antagonism of acupuncture analgesia in man by the narcotic antagonist naloxone', *Brain Research* 121. 36–37

Mayers, M. (1978) *A Systematic Approach to Nursing Care Plans* (Appleton-Century-Crofts, New York)

McCaffrey, M. (1968) *Cognition, Bodily Pain and Man/Environment Interactions* (University of California Student Store, Los Angeles)

McCaffrey, M., Ferrel, B. and Page, E. (1990) 'Nurses' knowledge of opioid analgesic drugs and psychological dependence', *Cancer Nursing* 13. 21–27

McCaffrey, M., Beebe, A. and Latham, J. (eds) (1994) *Pain: Clinical Manual for Nursing Practice* (Mosby, St Louis)

McCauley, J. D., Frank, R. G. and Callen, K. E. (1983) 'Hypnosis compared to relaxation in the outpatient management of chronic low back pain', *Archives of Physical Medicine and Rehabilitation* 64. 548–552

McClelland, J. L., Rumelhart, D. E. and PDP Research Group (1986) *Parallel Distributed Processing: Explorations in the Micro-structure of Cognition. Vol. 2. Psychological and Biological Models* (MIT Press, Cambridge MA)

McCormack, K. (1994) 'Non-steroidal anti-inflammatory drugs and spinal nociceptive processing', *Pain* 59. 9–43

McCracken, L. M. (1998) 'Learning to live with the pain: acceptance of pain predicts adjustment in persons with chronic pain', *Pain* 74. 21–27

McCusker, J. (1983) 'Where cancer patients die: an epidemiological study', *Public Health Reports* 98. 2. 170–176

McGrath, P. A. (1989) 'Evaluating a child's pain', *Journal of Pain and Symptom Management* 4. 4. 198–214

—— (1990) *Pain in Children: Nature, Assessment and Treatment* (The Guilford Press, New York)

McGrath, P. A. and de Veber, L. L. (1986) 'Helping children cope with painful procedures', *American Journal of Nursing* 86. 1,278–1,279

McGrath, P. A., Seifert, C. E., Speechley, K. N., Booth, J. C., Stitt, L. and Gibson, M. (1996) 'A new analogue scale for assessing children's pain: an initial validation study', *Pain* 64. 435–443

McGrath, P. J. (1990) 'Paediatric pain: a good start', *Pain* 41. 253–254

McGrath, P. J. and Unruh, A. M. (1994) 'Measurement and assessment of paediatric pain', in P. D. Wall and R. Melzack (eds) *Textbook of Pain* 3rd edn (Churchill Livingstone, Edinburgh)

McGrath, P. J., Johnson, G., Goodman, J. T., Schillinger, J., Dunn, J. and Chapman, J. (1985) 'The CHEOPS: a behavioural scale to measure postoperative pain in children', in H. L. Fields., R. Dubner and F. Cervero (eds) *Advances in Pain Research and Therapy* Vol. 9 (Raven Press, New York)

McGrath, P. J., Cunningham, S. J., Lascelles, M. and Humphreys, P. (1990) *Help Yourself: A Program for Treating Migraine Headaches* (University of Ottawa Press, Ottawa)

McGrath, P. J., Richie, J. and Unruh, A. (1993) 'Paediatric Pain', in D. Carroll and D. Bowsher (eds) (1993) *Pain: Management and Nursing Care* (Butterworth-Heinemann, Oxford)

McKenna, H. (1997) *Nursing Theories and Models* (Routledge, London)

Mead, G. H. (1934) *Mind, Self and Society from the Standpoint of a Social Behaviourist* (University of Chicago Press, Chicago)

Meadows, S. (1993) *The Child as Thinker: The Early Development and Acquisition of Cognition in Childhood* (Routledge, London)

Meerburg, G. (1993) 'Quality of life: a concept analysis', *Journal of Advanced Nursing* 18. 32–38

Melzack, R. (1975) 'The McGill Pain Questionnaire: major properties and scoring method', *Pain* 1. 277–299

—— (ed.) (1983) *Pain Measurement and Assessment* (Raven Press, New York)

—— (1987) 'The Short-form McGill Pain Questionnaire', *Pain* 30. 191–197

—— (1994) 'Folk medicine and the sensory modulation of pain', in P. D. Wall and R. Melzack (eds) *Textbook of Pain* 3rd edn (Churchill Livingstone, Edinburgh)

Melzack, R. and Katz, J. (1992) 'The McGill Pain Questionnaire: appraisal and current status', in D. Turk and R. Melzack (eds) *Handbook of Pain Assessment* (Guilford Press, New York)

Melzack, R. and Torgerson, W. S. (1971) 'On the language of pain', *Anesthesiology* 34. 50–59

Melzack, R. and Wall, P. D. (1965) 'Pain mechanisms. A new theory', *Science* 150. 971–979

—— (1996) *The Challenge of Pain* 2nd edn (Penguin, England)

Melzack, R., Ofiesh, J. G. and Mount, B. M. (1976) 'The Brompton Mixture effects on pain in cancer patients', *Canadian Medical Association Journal* 120. 435–438

Melzack, R., Stilwell, D. M. and Fox, E. J. (1977) 'Trigger points and acupressure points for pain: correlations and implications', *Pain* 3. 3–23

Melzack, R., Jeans, M. E., Stratford, J. G. and Monks, R. C. (1980) 'Ice massage and transcutaneous electrical stimulation: comparison of treatment for low back pain', *Pain* 9. 209–217

Melzack, R., Wall, P. D. and Ty, T. C. (1982) 'Acute pain in an emergency clinic: latency of onset and descriptor patterns', *Pain* 14. 33–43

Melzack, R., Abbott, F. V., Zackon, W., Mulder, D. S. and Davis, M. W. L. (1987) 'Pain on a surgical ward: a survey of the duration and intensity of pain and the effectiveness of medication', *Pain* 29. 67–72

Mendelson, G. (1984) 'Compensation, pain complaints and psychological disturbance', *Pain* 20. 169–175

——(1986) 'Chronic pain and compensation: a review', *Journal of Pain and Symptom Management* 1. 3. 135

Merskey, H. (1980) 'Some features of the history of the idea of chronic pain', *Pain* 9. 3–8

—— (1986) 'Classification of chronic pain: descriptions of chronic pain syndromes and definitions of pain terms', *Pain* (supplement 3) 1–225

Merton, R. K. (1957) 'The role set problems in sociological theory', *British Journal of Sociology* 8. 106–120

Meurier, C. E., Vincent, C. A. and Parmar, D. G. (1998) 'Perception of causes of omissions in the assessment of patients with chest pain', *Journal of Advanced Nursing* 28. 5. 1,012–1,019

Meyer, D. (1981) 'The effects of patients' representations of high blood pressure on behaviour in treatment' (Ph.D. Thesis, University of Wisconsin-Madison)

Meyer, R. A., Campbell, J. N. and Raja, S. N. (1994) 'Peripheral neural mechanisms of nociception', in P. D. Wall and R. Melzack (eds) *Textbook of Pain* 3rd edn (Churchill Livingstone, Edinburgh)

Meyer, W., Nichols, R. J. and Cortiella, J. (1997) 'Acetaminophen in the management of background pain in children post-burn', *Journal of Pain and Symptom Management* 13. 50–55

Miller, S. M. (1988) 'The interacting effects of coping styles and situational variables in gynaecologic settings: implications for research and treatment', *Journal of Psychosomatic Obstetrics and Gynaecology* 9. 23–34

Minghella, E. (1992) 'Depression and suicide', in J. Brooking, S. A. H. Ritter and B. Thomas (eds) *A Textbook of Psychiatric and Mental Health Nursing* (Churchill Livingstone, Edinburgh)

Miser, A. W., Davis, D. M., Hughes, C. S., Mulne, A. F. and Miser, J. S. (1983) 'Continuous subcutaneous infusion of morphine in children with cancer', *American Journal of Diseases of Children* 137. 383–385

Mishel, M. (1988) 'Uncertainty in illness', *Image: Journal of Nursing Scholarship* 20. 4. 225–232

Mobily, P., Herr, K. and Nicholson, A. (1994) 'Validation of cutaneous stimulation interventions for pain management', *International Journal of Nursing Studies* 31. 6. 533–544

Monga, T., Tan, G., Osterman, H. J., Monga, U. and Grabois, M. (1998) 'Sexuality and sexual adjustment of patients with chronic pain', *Disability and Rehabilitation* 20. 9. 317–329

Monks, R. and Merskey, H. (1984) 'Psychotropic drugs', in P. D. Wall and R. Melzack (eds) *Textbook of Pain* 1st edn (Churchill Livingstone, Edinburgh)

Moore, A., Collins, S., Carroll, D. and McQuay, H. (1997) 'Paracetamol with and without codeine in acute pain: a quantitative systematic review', *Pain* 70. 193–201

Moore, R. A. and McQuay, H. J. (1988) 'Single-patient data meta-analysis of 3,453 postoperative patients: oral tramadol versus placebo, codeine and combination analgesics', *Pain* 69. 287–294

Morley, S. (1993) 'Vivid memory for "everyday" pains', *Pain* 55. 55–62

Morley, S. and Wilkinson, L. (1995) 'The pain beliefs and perceptions inventory: a British replication', *Pain* 61. 427–433

Morley, S., Eccleston, C. and Williams, A. (1999) 'Systematic review and meta-analysis of randomized controlled trials of cognitive behaviour therapy and behaviour therapy for chronic pain in adults, excluding headache', *Pain* 80. 1–13

Morse, J. M. (1995) 'Exploring the theoretical basis of nursing using advanced techniques of concept analysis', *Advances in Nursing Science* 17. 3. 31–46

Morselli, P. I., Franco-Morselli, R. and Borsi, L. (1980) 'Clinical pharmacokinetics in newborns and infants. Age related differences and therapeutic implications', *Clinical Pharmacokinetics* 5. 485–527

Moscovici, S. (1984) 'The phenomenon of social representations', in R. M. Farr and S. Moscovici (eds) *Social Representations* (Cambridge University Press, Cambridge)

—— (1988) 'Notes towards a description of social representations', *European Journal of Social Psychology* 18. 211–250

Mountcastle, V. B. (1980) *Medical Physiology* (C. V. Mosby, St Louis)

Murry, T., Amundson, P. and Hollien, H. (1977) 'Acoustical characteristics of infant cries. Fundamental frequency', *Journal of Child Language* 4. 321–328

Nagy, S. (1998) 'A comparison of the effects of the patients' pain on nurses working in burns and neonatal intensive care units', *Journal of Advanced Nursing* 27. 335–340

Nash, R., Edwards, H. and Nebauer, M. (1993) 'Effect of attitudes, subjective norms and perceived control on nurses' intention to assess patients' pain', *Journal of Advanced Nursing* 18. 941–947

National Board of Health and Welfare Sweden (1987) *Att.forebygga sjukdomar I rorelseorganen* (Preventing musculoskeletal pain) (Socialstyrelsen, Stockholm)

National Institute of Mental Health (1982) *Television and Behaviour. Ten Years of Scientific Progress and Implications for the Eighties* Vol. 1 (US Government Printing Office, Washington DC)

Neher, A. (1991) 'Maslow's theory of motivation: a critique', *Journal of Humanistic Psychology* 31. 89–112

Nisbett, R. E., Caputo, C., Legant, P. and Marcek, J. (1973) 'Behaviour as seen by the actor and as seen by the observer', *Journal of Personality and Social Psychology* 27. 157–164

Noordenbos, W. (1959) *Pain* (Elsevier Press, Amsterdam)

O'Connor, L. (1995a) 'Pain assessment by patients and nurses, and nurses' notes on it, in early myocardial infarction, part 1', *Intensive and Critical Care Nursing* 11. 183–191

—— (1995b) 'Pain assessment by patients and nurses, and nurses' notes on it, in early myocardial infarction, part 2', *Intensive and Critical Care Nursing* 11. 283–292

O'Keefe, J. and Nadel, L. (1978) *The Hippocampus as a Cognitive Map* (Oxford University Press, New York)

Olness, K. and Gardner, G. (1988) *Hypnosis and Hypnotherapy with Children* (Grune and Stratton, New York)

Olson, D., Portnoy, J. and Lavee, Y. (1984) *FACES 111. Family Social Science* (University of Minnesota Press, St Paul MN)

Orem, D. E. (1995) *Nursing: Concepts of Practice* 5th edn (McGraw-Hill, New York)

Osborn, M. and Smith, J. A. (1998) 'The personal experience of chronic benign lower back pain: an interpretative phenomenological analysis', *British Journal of Health Psychology* 3. 65–83

Paediatric Vade Mecum (1993) (Edward Arnold, Birmingham)

Paice, J., Mahon, S. and Faut Callahan, M. (1991) 'Factors associated with adequate pain control in hospitalised post-surgical patients diagnosed with cancer', *Cancer Nursing* 14. 6. 298–305

Paice, J. A., Penn, R. D. and Shott, S. (1996) 'Intraspinal morphine for chronic pain: a retrospective, multicenter study', *Journal of Pain and Symptom Management* 11. 71–80

Paice, J. A., Winklemuller, W., Burchiel, K., Racz, G. B. and Prager, J. P. (1997) 'Clinical realities and economic considerations: efficacy of intrathecal pain therapy', *Journal of Pain and Symptom Management* 14. 3. 14–26

Paivio, A. (1991) 'Dual coding theory: retrospect and current status', *Canadian Journal of Psychology* 45. 255–287

Palmer, S. J. (1993) 'Care of sick children by parents: a meaningful role', *Journal of Advanced Nursing* 18. 185–191

Papez, J. W. (1937) 'A proposed mechanism of emotion', *Archives of Neurology and Psychiatry* 38. 725–743

Parsons, T. (1951) *The Social System* (Free Press, Glencoe IL)

Pavlov, I. P. (1927) *Conditioned Reflexes: An Investigation of the Physiological Activity of the Cerebral Cortex* (Dover, New York)

Pearce, C. (1993) 'Care of the dying', in D. Carroll and D. Bowsher (eds) *Pain: Management and Nursing Care* (Butterworth-Heinemann, Oxford)

Peck, J. R., Smith, T. W., Ward, J. and Milano, R. A. (1989) 'Disability and depression in rheumatoid arthritis: a multitrait multimethod investigation', *Arthritis and Rheumatism* 32. 9. 1,100–1,106

Pennebaker, J., Gonder-Frederick, L., Stewart, H., Elfman, L. and Skelton, J. (1981) 'Physical symptoms associated with blood pressure', *Psychophysiology* 19. 2. 201–210

Penner, L. and Rioux, S. (1995) 'The prosocial personality and memories of parents', Nags Head Invitation Conference on the Social Sciences, Highland Beach, June

Penson, J. and Fisher, R. (1991) *Palliative Care for People with Cancer* (Edward Arnold, London)

Perrin, E. C. and Gerrity, P. S. (1982) 'There's a demon in your belly: children's understanding of illness', *Pediatrics* 67. 841–849

Peters, J. L. and Large, R. G. (1990) 'A randomised controlled trial evaluating in and out patient pain management programmes', *Pain* 41. 283–293

Petrovitch-Bartell, N., Cowan, N. and Morse, P. A. (1982) 'Mothers' perceptions of infant distress vocalizations', *Journal of Speech and Hearing Research* 25. 371–376

Philips, H. C. (1988) 'Changing chronic pain experience', *Pain* 32. 165–172

Piaget, J. (1978) *The Development of Thought: Equilibration of Cognitive Structures* (Blackwell, Oxford)

—— (1983) 'Piaget's theory', in W. Kessen (ed.) *Handbook of Child Psychology* Vol. 1. Series ed. P. H. Mussen (previously published in 1970 in P. H. Mussen (ed.) *Carmichael's Manual of Child Psychology* 3rd edn, Vol. 1 (Wiley, New York))

Pilowski, I. (1990) 'The concept of abnormal illness behaviour', *Psychosomatics* 31. 2. 207–213

Pilowski, I. and Bassett, D. L. (1982) 'Pain and depression', *British Journal of Psychiatry* 141. 30–36

Pilowski, I. and Katsikitis, M. (1994) 'A classification of illness behaviour in pain clinic patients', *Pain* 57. 91–94

Pincus, T., Peace, S. and McLelland, A. (1993) 'Self-referential selective memory in pain patients', *British Journal of Clinical Psychology* 64. 331–344

Pither, C. E. (1989) 'Treatment of persistent pain', *British Medical Journal* 229. 12

Poole, K. (1998) 'The waiting game. A study of the psychological impact associated with diagnosing breast disease' (Ph.D. Thesis, School of Nursing Studies, University of Wales College of Medicine, Cardiff)

Portenoy, R. K. and Foley, K. M. (1986) 'Chronic use of opioid analgesics in non-malignant pain: a report of 38 cases', *Pain* 25. 171–176

Porter, F. L., Miller, R. H. and Marshall, R. E. (1986) 'Neonatal pain cries: effects of circumcision on acoustic features and perceived urgency', *Child Development* 57. 790

Price, D. D. (1988) *Psychological and Neurological Mechanisms of Pain* (Raven Press, New York)

Price, D. D. and Dubner, R. (1977) 'Mechanisms of first and second pain in peripheral and central nervous systems', *Journal of Investigative Dermatology* 69. 167–171

Procacci, P., Zoppi, M. and Maresca, M. (1994) 'Heart and vascular pain', in P. D. Wall. and R. Melzack (eds) *Textbook of Pain* 3rd edn (Churchill Livingstone, Edinburgh)

Rainville, P., Duncan, G. H., Price, D. D., Carrier, B. and Bushnell, M. C. (1997) 'Pain affect encoded in human anterior cingulate but not somatosensory cortex', *Science* 277. 5, 328. 968–971

Rang, H. P. and Bevan, D. A. (1994) 'Nociceptive peripheral neurons: cellular properties', in P. D. Wall. and R. Melzack (eds) *Textbook of Pain* 3rd edn (Churchill Livingstone, Edinburgh)

Rasmussen, S., Larsen, A. S., Thomsen, S. T. and Kehlet, H. (1998) 'Intra-articular glucocorticoid, bupivacaine and morphine reduces pain, inflammatory response and convalescence after arthroscopic meniscectomy', *Pain* 78. 131–134

Ready, L. B., Oden, R. and Chadwick, H. S. (1988) 'Development of an anesthesiology based postoperative pain management service', *Anesthesiology* 68. 100–116

Reid, G. J., Gilbert, C. A. and McGrath, P. J. (1998) 'The Pain Coping Questionnaire: preliminary validation', *Pain* 76. 83–96

Reid, S., Haugh, L. D., Hazard, R. G. and Tripathi, M. (1997) 'Occupational low back pain: recovery curves and factors associated with disability', *Journal of Occupational Rehabilitation* 7. 1–14

Revicky, D. A. (1989) 'Health related quality of life in the evaluation of medical therapy for chronic illness', *Journal of Family Practitioners* 29. 4. 377–380

Richardson, A. (1997) 'Cancer pain and its management', in V. N. Thomas (ed.) *Pain: Its Nature and Management* (Baillière Tindall, London)

Rigge, M. (1990) 'Pain', *Which? Way to Health* April. 66–68

Robinson, R. (1990) 'Personal narratives, social careers and medical courses: analysing life trajectories in autobiographies of people with multiple sclerosis', *Social Science and Medicine* 30. 1,173–1,186

Rogers, C. R. (1961) *On Becoming a Person: A Therapist's View of Psychotherapy* (Constable, London)

Rolfe, G. (1998) *Expanding Nursing Knowledge, Understanding and Researching Your Own Practice* (Butterworth-Heinemann, Oxford)

Romano, J. M. and Turner, J. A. (1985) 'Chronic pain and depression – does the evidence support a relationship?', *Psychological Bulletin* 97. 1. 18–34

Roop Moyer, S. M. and Howe, C. J. (1991) 'Pediatric pain intervention in the PACU', *Critical Care Nursing Clinics of North America* 3. 1. 49–57

Roper, N., Logan, N. and Tierney, A. (1990) *Elements of Nursing* 3rd edn (Churchill Livingstone, Edinburgh)

Rosch, E., Mervis, C. B., Gray, W. D., Johnson, D. M. and Boyes-Graem, P. (1976) 'Basic objects in natural categories', *Cognitive Psychology* 8. 382–439

Roscoe, A. K. and Myers, R. D. (1991) 'Hypothermia and feeding induced simultaneously in rats by perfusion of neuropeptide Y in preoptic area', *Pharmacology, Biochemistry and Behaviour* 39. 1,003–1,009

Rose, K. (1994) 'Patient isolation in chronic benign pain', *Nursing Standard* Sept., 8. 51

Rosenman, R. H. (1990) 'Type A behaviour patterns: a personal overview', *Journal of Social Behaviour and Personality* 5. 1–24

Rosensteil, A. K. and Keefe, F. J. (1983) 'The use of coping strategies in chronic low back pain patients: relationship to patient characteristics and current adjustment', *Pain* 17. 1. 33–44

Rosenthal, C. J., Marshall, V. W., Macpherson, A. S. and French, S. E. (1980) *Nurses, Patients and Families* (Croom Helm, London)

Ross, L., Amabile, T. and Steinmetz, J. (1977) 'Social rules, social control and biases in social perception processes', *Journal of Personality and Social Psychology* 35. 485–494

Ross, S. and Soltes, D. (1995) 'Heparin and haematoma: does ice make a difference?', *Journal of Advanced Nursing* 21. 3. 434–439

Rotter, J. (1966) 'Generalised expectancies for internal versus external control of reinforcement', *Psychological Monographs* 609. 80. 1. 1–28

Rowat, K. and Knafl, K. (1985) 'Living with chronic pain: the spouse's perspective', *Pain* 23. 259–272

Roy, C. (1985) 'The interactional perspective of pain behaviour in marriage', *International Journal of Family Therapy* 7. 71–83

—— (1988) 'The impact of chronic pain on marital partners. The system's perspective', in R. Dubner, G. Gebhart and M. Bon (eds) *Proceedings of the 5th World Congress on Pain* (Amsterdam, Elsevier)

—— (1989) *Chronic Pain and the Family: A Problem Centred Perspective* (Human Sciences Press, New York)

—— (1992) *The Social Context of the Chronic Pain Sufferer* (University of Toronto Press, Toronto)

—— (1996) *The Roy Adaptation Model. The Definitive Statement* (Appleton and Lange, Norwalk CT)

Roy, R. and Thomas, M. (1989) 'Nature of marital relations among chronic pain patients', *Contemporary Family Therapy* 11. 277–285

Royal College of Surgeons and College of Anaesthetists (1990) *Commission on the Provision of Surgical Services. Report of the Working Party on Pain after Surgery*, September

Rumelhart, D. E. (1980) 'Schemata: the building blocks of cognition', in R. J. Spiro *et al.* (eds) *Theoretical Issues in Reading Comprehension* (Lawrence Erlbaum, Hillsdale NJ)

Rumelhart, D. E. and Norman, D. A. (1983) *Representation in Memory: CHIP Technical Report (No.116)* (Center for Human Information Processing, University of California, San Diego CA). Reprinted in A. M. Aitkenhead and J. M. Slack (eds) (1985) *Issues in Cognitive Modelling* (Lawrence Erlbaum, Hillsdale NJ)

Russo, E. (1998) 'Cannabis for migraine treatment: the once and future prescription? An historical and scientific review', *Pain* 76. 3–8

Salvage, J. (1985) *The Politics of Nursing* (Butterworth-Heinemann, Oxford)

Salvage, J. and Kershaw, B. (eds) (1990) *Models of Nursing* 2 (Scutari Press, London)

Sanders, G. S. (1982) 'Social comparison and perceptions of health and illness', in G. S. Sanders and J. Suls (eds) *The Social Psychology of Health and Illness* (Lawrence Erlbaum, Hillsdale NJ)

Sanders, S. H. (1983) 'Automated vs. self help monitoring of "up-time" in chronic low back pain patients: a comparative study', *Pain* 15. 399–405

Sartorious, N. (1991) 'Kvaliteta zivota (quality of life)', in B. Vrhovac, I. Bakran, M. Granic, B. Jaksic, B. Lanar and B. Bvucelic (eds) *Interna Medicina* Vol. 1 (Naprijed Zagreb) (in Croatian)

Saunders, C. (ed.) (1978) *The Management of Terminal Disease* (Edward Arnold, London)

—— (1994) 'Pain and impending death', in P. D. Wall and R. Melzack (eds) *Textbook of Pain* 3rd edn (Churchill Livingstone, Edinburgh)

Savendra, M. C., Gibbons, P., Tesler, M., Ward, J. and Wegner, C. (1982) 'How do children describe pain? A tentative assessment', *Pain* 14. 95–104

Savendra, M. C., Holzemer, W. L., Tesler, M. D. and Wilkie, D. J. (1993) 'Assessment of postoperation pain in children and adolescents using the Adolescent Pediatric Pain Tool', *Nursing Research* 42. 1. 5–9

Scadding, J. W. (1994) 'Peripheral neuropathies', in P. D. Wall and R. Melzack (eds) *Textbook of Pain* 3rd edn (Churchill Livingstone, Edinburgh)

Schachter, S. and Singer, J. E. (1962) 'Cognitive, social and physiological determinants of emotional state', *Psychological Review* 69. 379–399

Schank, R. C. and Abelson, R. P. (1977) *Scripts, Plans, Goals and Understanding* (Lawrence Erlbaum, Hillsdale NJ)

Schechter, N. L., Allen, D. A. and Hanson, K. (1986) 'Status of pediatric pain control: a comparison of hospital analgesic usage in children and adults', *Pediatrics* 77. 11–15

Schechter, N. L., Berrien, F. B. and Katz, S. M. (1988) 'The use of patient controlled analgesia in adolescents with sickle cell pain crisis: a preliminary report', *Journal of Pain and Symptom Management* 3. 109–113

Schechter, N. L., Weisman, S. J., Rosenblum, M., Beck, A., Altman, A., Quinn, J. and Conrad, P. F. (1990) 'Sedation for pain procedures in children with cancer using the fentanyl lollipop: a preliminary report', in D. C. Tyler and E. J. Krane (eds) *Advances in Pain Research Therapy* Vol. 15 (Raven Press, New York)

Schmitt, P. (1985) 'Rehabilitation of chronic pain: principles for rehabilitation counselling', *Rehabilitation Counselling Bulletin* 28. 15–27

Schoenen, J. and Maertens de Noordhout, A. (1994) 'Headache', in P. D. Wall and R. Melzack (eds) *Textbook of Pain* 3rd edn (Churchill Livingstone, Edinburgh)

Schofield, P. and Davis, B. (1998) 'Sensory deprivation and chronic pain: a review of the literature', *Disability and Rehabilitation* 20. 10. 357–366

Schutz, W. C. (1960) *FIRO: A Three Dimensional Theory of Interpersonal Behaviour* (Holt, Rinehart and Winston, New York)

Scott, D. S. and Barber, T. X. (1977) 'Cognitive control of pain: effects of multiple cognitive strategies', *Psychology Record* 2. 373–383

Sear, J. W., Hand, C. W., Moore, R. A. and McQuay, H. J. (1989) 'Studies on morphine disposition: influence of renal failure on the kinetics of morphine and its metabolites', *British Journal of Anaesthesia* 62. 28–32

Seers, C. J. (1987) 'Pain, anxiety and recovery in patients undergoing surgery' (Ph.D. Thesis, University of London)

Seers, K. (1987) 'Perception of pain', *Nursing Times* 83. 48. 37–39

Seers, K. and Carroll, D. (1998) 'Relaxation techniques for acute pain management: a systematic review', *Journal of Advanced Nursing* 27. 466–475

Seers, K. and Davis, P. (1993) 'Pain in the nursing curriculum', in D. Carroll and D. Bowsher (eds) *Pain: Management and Nursing Care* (Butter-worth-Heinemann, Oxford)

Seligman, M. E. P. (1975) *Helplessness: On Depression, Development and Death* (W. H. Freeman, San Francisco)

Selye, H. (1956) *The Stress of Life* (McGraw-Hill, New York)

Shanfield, S., Heiman, E., Cope, N. and Jones, J. (1979) 'Pain and the marital relationship: psychiatric distress', *Pain* 7. 343–351

Sheikh, K. (1987) 'Occupational injury, chronic low back pain and return to work', *Public Health* 101. 6. 417–425

Shere, C. L., O'Sullivan, J. A., Doleys, P. and Canan, B. (1986) 'The effect of two sites of high frequency vibration on cutaneous pain threshold', *Pain* 25. 133–138

Simmonds, M. J., Kumar, S. and Lechelt, E. (1998) 'Psychosocial factors in disabling low back pain: causes or consequences?', *Disability and Rehabilitation* 18. 4. 161–168

Sims, S. (1986) 'Slow stroke back massage for cancer patients', *Nursing Times* 82. 47–50

Sindhu, F. (1996) 'Are non-pharmacological nursing interventions for the management of pain effective? A meta-analysis', *Journal of Advanced Nursing* 24. 1,152–1,159

Skevington, S. M. (1986) 'Psychological aspects of pain in rheumatoid arthritis: a review', *Social Science and Medicine* 23. 6. 567–575

—— (1990) 'A standardised scale to measure beliefs about controlling pain (The BPCQ): a preliminary study', *Psychology and Health* 4. 221–232

—— (1993) 'Depression and causal attributions in the early stages of a chronic painful disease: a longitudinal study of early sinovitis', *Psychology and Health* 8. 51–64

—— (1995) *Psychology of Pain* (John Wiley, Chichester)

—— (1998) 'Investigating the relationship between pain and discomfort and quality of life, using the WHOQOL', *Pain* 76. 395–406

Skinner, B. F. (1938) *The Behaviour of Organisms* (Appleton-Century-Crofts, New York)

—— (1953) *Science and Human Behaviour* (Macmillan, New York)

—— (1971) *Beyond Freedom and Dignity* (Bantam, New York)

Sloan, P. A. (1986) 'Nitrous oxide/oxygen analgesia in palliative care', *Journal of Palliative Care* 2. 43–48

Smith, J. L. and Noon, J. (1998) 'Obstetric measurement of mood change induced by contemporary music', *Journal of Psychiatric and Mental Health Nursing* 5. 5. 403–408

Smooha, S. (1985) 'Ethnic groups', in A. Kuper and J. Kuper (eds) *The Social Science Encyclopaedia* (Routledge and Kegan Paul, London)

Snell, C. C., Fothergill-Bourbonnais, F. and Durocher-Hendricks, S. (1997) 'Patient controlled analgesia and intramuscular injections: a comparison of pain experiences and postoperative outcomes', *Journal of Advanced Nursing* 25. 681–690

Snelling, J. (1994) 'The effect of chronic pain on the family unit', *Journal of Advanced Nursing* 19. 543–551

Snyder, S. (1980) 'Brain peptides as neurotransmitters', *Science* 209. 976–983

Sofaer, B. (1984) 'The effect of focused education for nursing teams on postoperative pain of patients' (Ph.D. Thesis, University of Edinburgh)

—— (1998) *Pain: Principles Practice and Patients* (Stanley Thornes, Cheltenham)

Soper, W. Y. and Melzack, R. (1982) 'Stimulation-produced analgesia: evidence for somatotopic organisation in the midbrain', *Brain Research* 51. 307–311

Spanos, N. P., Carmanico, S. J. and Ellis, J. A. (1994) 'Hypnotic Analgesia', in P. D. Wall and R. Melzack (eds) *Textbook of Pain* 3rd edn (Churchill Livingstone, Edinburgh)

Spielberger, C. (1966) *Anxiety and Behaviour* (Academic Press, New York)

Spielberger, C., Gorsuch, L. and Lushene, R. (1970) *The State Trait Anxiety Inventory* (Oxford Psychologists Press, Oxford)

Spielberger, C., Gorsuch, L., Lushene, R., Vagg, P. and Jacobs, G. (1983) *STAI Manual for the State-Trait Anxiety Inventory* (Consulting Psychologists Press, Palo Alto)

Stannard, C. (ed.) (1998) 'GMC performance procedures in pain management', *Newsletter of the Pain Society* Autumn, 1. 4.

Stauffer, J. D. (1987) 'Antidepressants and chronic pain', *Journal of Family Practice* 25. 167–170

Sternbach, R. A. (1968) *Pain. A Psychophysiological Analysis* (Academic Press, New York)

—— (1974) 'Varieties of pain games', in J. Bonica (ed.) *Advances in Neurology* Vol. 4 (Raven Press, New York)

Sternbach, R. A. and Tursky, B. (1965) 'Ethnic differences among housewives in psycho-physiological and skin responses to electric shock', *Psychophysiology* 1. 217–218

Stevens, B. (1990) 'Development and testing of a paediatric pain management sheet', *Paediatric Nursing* 16. 543–548

Stevenson, C. (1995) 'Aromatherapy', in D. Rankin-Box (ed.) *The Nurses' Handbook of Complementary Therapies* (Churchill Livingstone, Edinburgh)

Stockwell, F. (1972) *The Unpopular Patient*, Royal College of Nursing Research Project Series 1, No. 2 (Royal College of Nursing, London)

Storms, M. D. (1973) 'Videotape and the attribution process: reversing actors' and observers' points of view', *Journal of Personality and Social Psychology* 27. 165–175

Strauss, A., Schatzman, L., Ehrlich, D., Bucher, R. and Sabshin, M. (1963) 'The hospital and its negotiated order', in E. Friedson (ed.) *The Hospital in Modern Society* (Collier-Macmillan, London)

Sullivan, M. J. L., Stanish, W., Waite, H., Sullivan, M. and Tripp, D. A. (1998) 'Catastrophizing, pain and disability in patients with soft-tissue injuries', *Pain* 77. 253–260

Swerdlow, M. (1984) 'Anticonvulsant drugs and chronic pain', *Clinical Neuropharmacology* 7. 51–82

Szasz, T. (1973) *The Manufacture of Madness* (Paladin, London)

Taenzer, P. A. (1983) 'Self control of postoperative pain: effects of hypnosis and waking suggestion' (Ph.D. Thesis, McGill University, Montreal)

Tait, R. C. and Chibnall, J. T. (1998) 'Attitude profiles and the clinical status in patients with chronic pain', *Pain* 78. 49–57

Tajfel, H. (1978) *Differentiation Between Social Groups: Studies in the Social Psychology of Intergroup Relations* (Academic Press, London).

—— (1991) *Social Identity and Intergroup Relations* (Cambridge, Cambridge University Press)

Tarter, R. E., Erb, S., Biller, P. A., Switala, J. and van Thiel, D. H. (1988) 'The quality of life following liver transplantation', *Gastro-enterology Clinics of North America* 17. 1. 207–217

Taylor, C. B., Zlutnick, S. I., Corley, M. J. and Flora, J. (1980) 'The effects of detoxification, relaxation, and brief supportive therapy on chronic pain', *Pain* 8. 319–329

Taylor, P. (1983) 'Postoperative pain in toddler and preschool age children', *Maternal and Child Nursing* 12. 35–50

Tempest, S. (1993) 'The pharmacology of analgesics', in D. Carroll and D. Bowsher (eds) *Pain: Management and Nursing Care* (Butterworth-Heinemann, Oxford)

Thomas, V. N. (ed.) (1997) *Pain: Its Nature and Management* (Baillière Tindall, London)

Thompson, I. E., Melia, K. M. and Boyd, K. M. (1994) *Nursing Ethics* 3rd edn (Churchill Livingstone, Edinburgh)

Thorndyke, E. L. (1931) *Human Learning* (Century, New York)

Toates, F. (1986) *Biological Foundations of Behaviour* (Open University Press, Milton Keynes)

Tolman, E. C. (1932) *Purposive Behaviour in Animal and Man* (Century, New York)

—— (1948) 'Cognitive maps in rats and men', *The Psychological Review* 55. 189–208

Tomlinson, A. (1991) 'Leisure and the quality of life: themes and issues', *Leisure Studies Association* 42

Toomey, T. C., Mann, J. D., Abashian, S. and Thompson Pope, S. (1991) 'Relationship between perceived self control of pain, pain description and functioning', *Pain* 45. 129–133

Torres, F. and Anderson, C. (1985) 'The normal EEG of the human', *Journal of Clinical Neurophysiology* 2. 89–103

Towell, T. (1999) 'Clinical effectiveness in pain management for patients following coronary artery bypass grafts' (M.Phil. Thesis, School of Nursing, University of Wales College of Medicine, Cardiff)

Treede, R. D., Kenshalo, D. R., Gracely, R. H. and Jones, A. K. P. (1999) 'The cortical representation of pain', *Pain* 79. 105–111

Trief, P. and Stein, N. (1985) 'Pending litigation and rehabilitation outcome of chronic back pain', *Archives of Physical Medicine and Rehabilitation* 66. 95–99

Trounce, J. (1997) *Clinical Pharmacology for Nurses* (Churchill Livingstone, Edinburgh)

Tunks, E. (1990) 'Chronic pain and the occupational role Part 1', in E. Tunks, A. Bellissimo and R. Roy (eds) *Chronic Pain: Psychosocial Factors in Rehabilitation* 2nd edn (Krieger, Melbourne FL)

Turk, D. C. and Fernandez, E. (1991) 'Pain: a cognitive-behavioural perspective', in M Watson (ed.) *Cancer Patient Care Psychosocial Treatment Methods* (BPS Books, Cambridge)

Turk, D. C. and Flor, H. (1987) 'Pain behaviours: the utility and limitations of the pain behaviour construct', *Pain* 31. 277–295

Turk, D. C. and Genest, M. (1979) 'Regulation of pain: the application of cognitive and behavioural techniques for prevention and remediation', in P. C. Kendall and S. D. Hollon (eds) *Cognitive-Behavioural Interventions Theory Research and Procedures* (Academic Press, New York)

Turk, D. C. and Melzack, R. (eds) (1992) *Handbook of Pain Assessment* (Guilford Press, New York)

Turk, D. C. and Rudy, T. E. (1986) 'Assessment of cognitive factors in chronic pain: a worthwhile enterprise', *Journal of Consulting and Clinical Psychology* 56. 2. 233–238

—— (1990) 'The robustness of an empirically derived taxonomy of chronic pain patients', *Pain* 43. 27–35

Turk, D. C., Meichenbaum, D. and Genest, M. (1983) *Pain and Behavioural Medicine* (Guilford Press, New York)

Turk, D. C., Okifuji, A. and Scharff, L. (1995) 'Chronic pain and depression: role of perceived impact and perceived control in different age cohorts', *Pain* 61. 93–101

Turner, J. A. and Chapman, C. R. (1982a) 'Psychological interventions for chronic pain: a critical review. 1. Relaxation training and biofeedback', *Pain* 12. 1–12

—— (1982b) 'Psychological interventions for chronic pain: a critical review. 2. Operant conditioning, hypnosis, and cognitive-behavioural therapy', *Pain* 12. 23–46

Turner, J. and Romano, J. M. (1984) 'Evaluating psychologic interventions for chronic pain: issues and recent developments', in C. Benedetti,

C. R. Chapman and G. Moricca (eds) *Advances in Pain Research and Therapy* Vol. 7 (Raven Press, New York)

Turner, J. C., Oakes, P. and McGarty, C. (1993) 'Self and collective: cognition and social context', *Personality and Psychology Bulletin* 20. 454–463

Turner, J. G., Clark, A. J., Gauthier, D. K. and Williams, M. (1998) 'The effect of therapeutic touch on pain and anxiety in burn patients', *Journal of Advanced Nursing* 28. 10–20

Turner, R. H. (1962) 'Role-taking: process versus conformity', in A. M. Rose (ed.) *Human Behaviour and Social Processes* (Routledge and Kegan Paul, London)

Twycross, A. and Lack, S. A. (1990) *Therapeutics in Terminal Cancer* (Churchill Livingstone, Edinburgh)

Twycross, A., Moriarty, A. and Betts, T. (1998) *Paediatric Pain Management: A Multidisciplinary Approach* (Radcliffe Medical Press, Oxford)

Twycross, R. G. (1979) 'The Brompton Cocktail', in J. J. Bonica and V. Ventafridda (eds) *Advances in Pain Research and Therapy* Vol. 2 (Raven Press, New York)

Tyrer, S. (1992) 'Psychiatric assessment of chronic pain', *British Journal of Psychiatry* 160. 733–741

UKCC (1992a) 'Code of Practice', *United Kingdom Central Council for Nursing, Midwifery and Health Visiting* (UKCC, London)

—— (1992b) 'Standards for the administration of medicines for nurses', *United Kingdom Central Council for Nursing, Midwifery and Health Visiting* (UKCC, London)

Unruh, A., McGrath, P. J., Cunningham, S. J. and Humphreys, P. (1983) 'Children's drawing of their pain', *Pain* 17. 385–392

Valente, S. M. (1991) 'Using hypnosis with children for pain management', *Oncology Nursing Forum* 18. 4. 699–704

Van Tulder, M. W., Koes, B. W. and Bouter, L. M. (1995) 'A cost of illness study of low back pain in the Netherlands', *Pain* 62. 233–240

Varni, J. W., Thompson, K. L. and Hanson, V. (1987) 'The Varni/Thompson Pediatric Questionnaire: I. Chronic musculoskeletal pain in juvenile rheumatoid arthritis', *Pain* 28. 27–38

Vaughan, H. E. (1975) 'Electrophysiologic analysis of regional cortical maturation', *Biological Psychiatry* 10. 513–526

Verhaak, P. F. M., Kerssens, J. J., Dekker, J., Marjolijn, J. S. and Bensing, J. M. (1998) 'Prevalence of chronic benign pain disorder among adults: a review of the literature', *Pain* 77. 231–239

Victor, J. S., McEnvoy, B., Becker, M. H. and Rosenstock, I. M. (1986) 'Self-efficacy', *Health Education Quarterly* 13. 73–91

Vlaeyen, J. W. S., Van Eek, H., Groenman, N. H. and Schuerman, J. A. (1987) 'Dimensions and components of observed chronic pain behaviour', *Pain* 31. 65–75

Vygotsky, L. S. (1962) *Thought and Language* (MIT Press, Cambridge MA)

—— (1986) *Thought and Language* new edn ed. A. Kozulin (MIT Press, Cambridge MA)

Wachtel, P. (1977) *Psychoanalysis and Behaviour Therapy: Toward an Integration* (New York, Basic Books)

Waddell, G. (1996) 'Low back pain: a twentieth-century health care enigma', *Spine* 21. 2,820–2,825

Walding, M. (1991) 'Pain, anxiety and powerlessness', *Journal of Advanced Nursing* 16. 388–397

Walker, J. and Sofaer, B. (1998) 'Predictors of psychological distress in chronic pain patients', *Journal of Advanced Nursing* 27. 320–326

Walker, J., Akinsanya, J., Davis, B. and Marcer, D. (1989) 'The nursing management of patients with pain in the community: a theoretical framework', *Journal of Advanced Nursing* 14. 240–247

—— (1990) 'The nursing management of patients with pain in the community: study and recommendations', *Journal of Advanced Nursing* 15. 1,114–1,116

Wall, P. D. (1989) 'Introduction', in P. D. Wall and R. Melzack (eds) *Textbook of Pain* 2nd edn (Churchill Livingstone, Edinburgh)

Wall, P. D. and Jones, M. (1991) *Defeating Pain. The War against the Silent Epidemic* (Plenum, New York)

Wall, P. D. and Sweet, W. H. (1967) 'Temporary abolition of pain', *Science* 155. 108–109

Wallston, K. A. (1989) 'Control in chronic illness', paper presented to the International Conference on Health Psychology, Cardiff

Watson, D. and Clark, L. A. (1992) 'Affects separable and inseparable: on the hierarchical arrangement of the negative affects', *Journal of Personality and Social Psychology* 62. 489–505

Watson, J. B. and Rayner, R. (1920) 'Conditioned emotional reactions', *Journal of Experimental Psychology* 3. 1–14

Watt-Watson, J. (1987) 'Nurses' knowledge of pain issues: a survey', *Journal of Pain Symptom Management* 2. 4. 207–211

Weddell, G. (1955) 'Somesthesis and the chemical senses', *Annual Review of Psychology* 6. 119

Weiner, B. (1985) 'An attributional theory of achievement, motivation and emotion', *Psychological Review* 92. 548–573

Weisenberg, M. (1994) 'Cognitive aspects of pain', in P. D. Wall and R. Melzack (eds) *Textbook of Pain* 3rd edn (Churchill Livingstone, Edinburgh)

Weisenberg, M., Raz, T. and Hener, T. (1998) 'The influence of film induced mood on pain perception', *Pain* 76. 365–375

Weissman, D. E. and Dahl, J. L. (1990) 'Attitudes about cancer pain: a survey of Wisconsin's first year medical students', *Journal of Pain and Symptom Management* 5. 6. 345–349

Westen, D. (1996) *Psychology: Mind, Brain and Culture* (Wiley, New York)

Wheatley, R. G., Madej, T. H., Jackson, I. J. B. and Hunter, D. (1991) 'The first year's experience of an acute pain service', *British Journal of Anaesthesia* 67. 353–359

Williams, A. (1985) *Quality of Life Adjusted Years and Coronary Artery Bypass Grafting* (Department of Health and Social Security, London)

Williams, A. Cde C., Nicholas, M. K., Richardson, P. H., Pither, C. E., Justins, D. M., Chamberlain, J. H., Harding, J. R., Ralphs, J A., Jones, S C., Dieudonne, I., Featherstone, J. D., Hodgson, D. R., Ridout, K. L. and Shannon, E. M. (1993) 'Evaluation of a cognitive behavioural programme for rehabilitating patients with chronic pain', *British Journal of General Practice* 43. 513–518

Williams, D. and Page, M. M. (1989) 'A multi-dimensional measure of Maslow's hierarchy of needs', *Journal of Research in Personality* 23. 192–213

Williams, D. A., Robinson, M. E. and Geisser, M. E. (1994) 'Pain beliefs: assessment and utility', *Pain* 59. 71–78

Williams, D. A., Urban, B., Keefe, F., Shutty, M. S. and France, R. (1995) 'Cluster analysis of pain patients' responses to the SCL-90R', *Pain* 61. 81–91

Wills, T. A. (1991) 'Similarity and self esteem in downward comparison', in J. Suls and T. A. Wills (eds) *Social Comparison: Contemporary Theory and Research* (Lawrence Erlbaum, Hillsdale NJ)

Wilson-Barnett, J. (1997) 'Patient teaching: a pain management strategy', in V. N. Thomas (ed.) *Pain: Its Nature and Management* (Baillière Tindall, London)

Winkelmuller, M. and Winkelmuller, W. (1996) 'Long-term effects of continuous intrathecal opioid treatment in chronic pain of nonmalignant etiology', *Journal of Neurological Surgery* 85. 458–467

Wolff, P. H. (1974) 'Active language: the natural history of crying and other vocalisations in early infancy', in L. J. Stone., H. T. Smith and L. B. Murphy (eds) *The Competent Infant* (Tavistock, London)

Wolke, D. (1987) 'Environmental and developmental neonatology', *Journal of Reproductive and Infant Psychology* 5. 17

Wong, D. L. and Baker, C. M. (1988) 'Pain in children: comparison of assessment scales', *Pediatric Nursing* 14. 1. 9–17

Wood, D. J., Bruner, J. S. and Ross, G. (1976) 'The role of tutoring in problem solving', *Journal of Child Psychology and Psychiatry* 17. 2. 89–100

Woodrow, R. M., Friedman, G. D., Siegelaub, A. B. and Cohen, M. F. (1972) 'Pain tolerance: differences according to age, sex and race', *Psychosomatic Medicine* 34. 548–556

Woolf, C. J. and Thompson, J. W. (1994) 'Stimulation-induced analgesia: transcutaneous electrical nerve stimulation (TENS) and vibration', in P. D. Wall and R. Melzack (eds) *Textbook of Pain* 3rd edn (Churchill Livingstone, Edinburgh)

Woolf, C. J. and Wall, P. D. (1983) 'Endogenous opioid peptides and pain mechanisms: a complex relationship', *Nature* 306. 739–740

World Health Organisation (1980) *International Classification of Impairments, Disabilities and Handicaps* (World Health Organisation, Geneva)

—— (1996) *Cancer Pain Relief*, WHO Technical Report Series (World Health Organisation, Geneva)

Yaksh, T. L. (ed.) (1986) *Spinal Afferent Processing* (Plenum, New York)

Yaksh, T. L. and Malmberg, A. B. (1994) 'Central pharmacology of nociceptive transmission', in P. D. Wall and R. Melzack (eds) *Textbook of Pain* 3rd edn (Churchill Livingstone, Edinburgh)

Yamamoto, T. and Nozaki-Taguchi, N. (1997) 'Analysis of the roles of cyclooxygenase (COX-1 and COX-2)', in *Spinal Nociceptive Transmission. Proceedings of the 8th World Congress in Pain Research and Management* Vol. 8 (IASP Press, Seattle)

Yerkes, R. M. and Dodson, J. D. (1908) 'The relation of the strength of stimulus to rapidity of habit formation', *Journal of Comparative Neurological Psychology* 18. 459–482

Zalon, M. L. (1993) 'Nurses' assessment of postoperative patients' pain', *Pain* 54. 329–334

Zborowski, M. (1952) 'Cultural components in responses to pain', *Journal of Social Issues* 8. 16–30

Zimmerman, L., Pozehl, B. and Duncan, K. (1989) 'Effects of music in patients who had chronic cancer pain', *Western Journal of Nursing Research* 11. 3. 298–309

Zucker, T. P., Flesche, C. W., Germing, U., Schroter, S., Willers, R., Wolf, H. H. and Heyll, A. (1998) 'Patient-controlled versus staff-controlled analgesia with pethidine after allogeneic bone marrow transplantation', *Pain* 75. 305–312

Index